#KickingCancer
My Battle Told Through Social Media

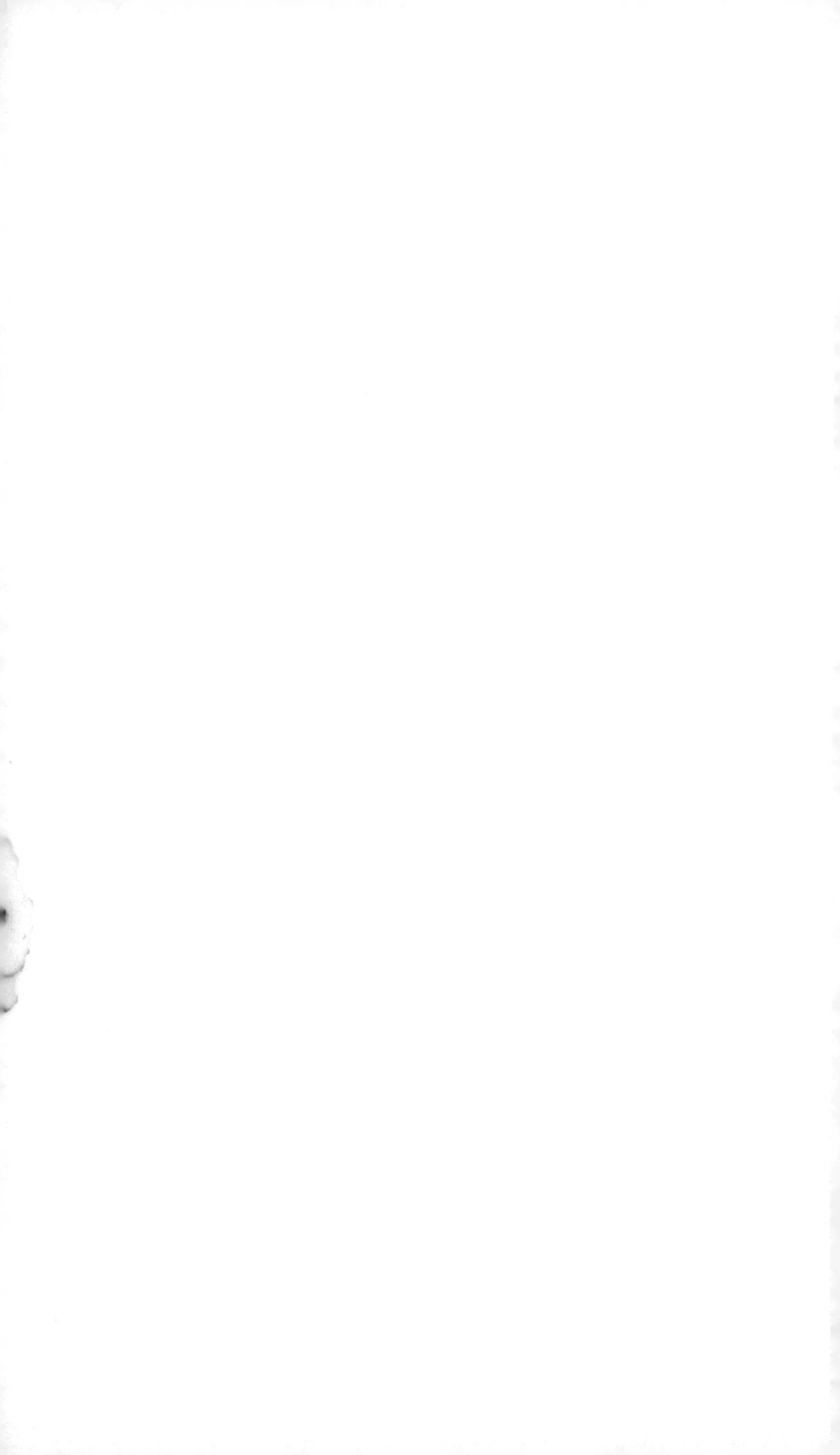

#KickingCancer
My Battle Told Through Social Media

Eric Glynn

Cover design by Double Seven Enterprise and Allie Benz
Interior design and typsetting by Double Seven Enterprise

ISBN: 1508837414
ISBN 13: 9781508837411

Just like the rising sun,
Thank you goes out to everyone

9-3-14: The Day of My Diagnosis

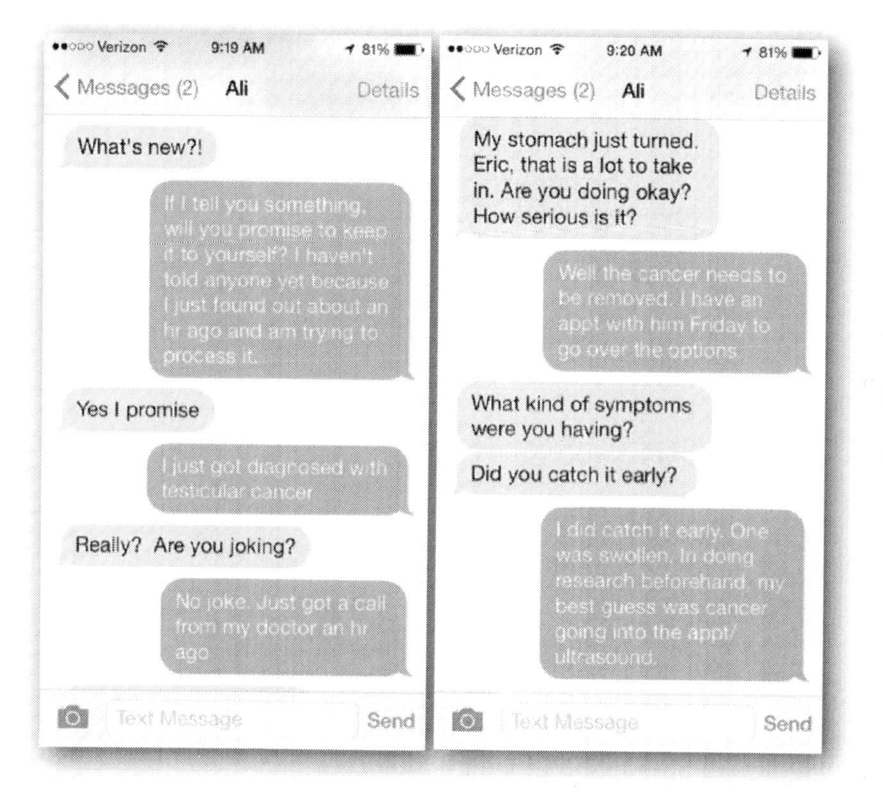

My First Blog Post: The Past Week...

by ERIC GLYNN, Wednesday, September 8, 2014

Hey all. So, this last week has been one of taking a lot of tests, asking a lot of questions and getting a lot of tough diagnoses. I wanted to get the full scope of what I'm about to go through before I shared with everyone.

So last Wednesday I had some tests run, including two ultrasounds. At about 6:30 p.m. that night, I got a call from my urologist telling me I have testicular cancer, and that we have to have surgery as soon as possible. I scheduled an appointment for that Friday to meet and pick a a surgery date, review the blood work that was taken, and do some Q&A.

Three days ago, Friday, I came in for that follow-up appointment. The blood work came back very poor. For a couple of the tests, the numbers that show up (that's as scientific as I go) are supposed to be less than 10, but for me came up in the thousands. This led the urologist to believe that the cancer spread, and that I should have a CT scan scheduled.

We scheduled surgery for Wednesday (two days from now) because that needs to be removed for sure, and that we'd face whatever other cancer we discover as it comes.

So, finally, today. This morning I went in and got the CT scan on my brain, chest, stomach and pelvis. About an hour ago, I got a call from the radiologist. The cancer spread to my left kidney and lymph nodes, and it is too large to operate on in its current state. The only option is to do chemotherapy and hopefully shrink the cancer small enough to where they will be able to surgically remove it. He referred me to the University of Southern California (USC) here in Los Angeles, as they're doing some breakthrough things with cancer treatment. So after my surgery on Wednesday, I will make my first appointment with the USC oncology department and find out exactly what type of chemo I will need to undertake to get the cancer to a state where I can have another surgery.

So, being that I just moved to California from Minnesota two weeks ago, my mom convinced me she needs to come out here for the surgery, so she's coming in tomorrow morning and hasn't booked a ticket home yet. She'll be my nurse :) … and though I only know a couple people — Tony and Theresa Borszcz and RJ Root — here in Huntington Beach, they are of the highest quality, and will absolutely help and support me when family isn't around. I'm sure any of those three would be more than happy to ice my junk after my surgery, am I right guys???

So, I made this blog thing so people who would like to can follow along. I guess if you've plugged in your email you'll get notifications when I update, and you can post comments and stuff. It'll be way easier for me to do it this way over calls, texts, emails, etc.

I've gotten so much love in so many ways already and it's been truly amazing. I know you all have my back like crazy, and I'll be good about keeping this thing updated so you all don't feel neglected as I go through this. If you know me at all, you know I'm doing okay. I can see humor in everything, no matter how shitty. For instance, my catchphrase for this first phase is, "I'm going to kick cancer in the balls," and I actually named the testicular tumor "Ball Bunyan" ... a shout out to Minnesota's Paul Bunyan. If you believe in prayer, pray for me. If you just pull me into your thoughts sometimes, that's great too. I know I'm not by myself as I kick start all this stuff.

Next time I post I'll probably be all drugged up from surgery, so forgive any typing errors or random tangents. If I start complaining about my fantasy football team or LA traffic just skip over those parts...

Favorite Comments

Hey Eric, cancer can be beat!! It's a tough road but hang in there. Thoughts and prayers are with you. Keep your sense of humor - it will help you get through this!
—Mary Jo Jasper, September 8, 2014

John just stopped by. I literally sobbed, I was so touched. He brought a bottle of JD for me to bring to you in CA tomorrow, but I'm doing carry on, so only 3 ounces allowed. So John, Alan and I drank it down to 3 ounces. Cheers!
—Eric's Mom

Wow Glynn! You sure are handling this in true Eric Glynn fashion :) I'll be thinking of you often and rooting for you in your ball kicking quest. Hang in there!!
—Kelly Bundy, September 8, 2014

Preface

Rewind nine months. December 2013. 27 years old. Making a very comfortable six-figure salary in sales for a software company. I was a bachelor with a disposable income living in fun little Uptown Minneapolis, Minnesota… just 20 minutes north of the suburb I grew up in. Amazing family and friends all over the state. Fancy apartment overlooking Lake Calhoun. Badass, right? Nope. I was so sick of Minnesota. We were right in the middle of a winter that turned out to be the coldest average temperature in Minnesota since World War II. That was the last straw for me. I just wasn't built for subzero temperatures, snow, ice… unlike everyone else in Minnesota, snowboarding, skiing, ice skating and ice fishing sound like the most horrible, cold, lame activities I could think of. Just not a Minnesota boy.

I actually had already lived in California once and loved it. I lived in San Diego for a year and a half, but got homesick. And this was the winter I came home to. Thanks for reminding me why I left in the first place, Minnesota.

I had recently started a new job with a software company, which meant eight weeks of training in Colorado between

September and November 2013. Which also meant room service, fancy dinners, drinking... aaaaand putting on a bunch of weight.

So I'm at a Christmas Eve gathering at my grandma's house, upset with my current physical plumpness and fussy about another Minnesota winter. Out of absolutely nowhere as I'm putting on my jacket to leave, my grandma pulls me aside and asks me if I have diabetes. I didn't connect the dots right away. I kinda laughed and said no... but then after a couple minutes of my drive home I was like... she asked me if I have diabetes because I look like an unhealthy fat ass!

She was the first one to call me out on it. It jarred me that night. And I decided I'd follow suit with what millions of others do (and usually fail at)... come January 1st, I'm going to get in shape.

Up to that point, my will to exercise and practice any type of food portion control had been poor. Lazy. But January 1, 2014, I started kicking ass. Literally every day from January to April, whether I was at home or on the road for work, I would get on an elliptical. In April, I started mixing weight lifting in with the cardio. I was killing it.

By July 2014, I had lost 60 pounds and was pure muscle. No steroids, no diet pills... just hard work in the gym and the kitchen. I had never been stronger, never had that much stamina. Inside and out, I was feeling great. I started an Instagram account to track my progress, to motivate others, and to perhaps gain a following in case I were to someday make a career change and do something in fitness or nutrition.

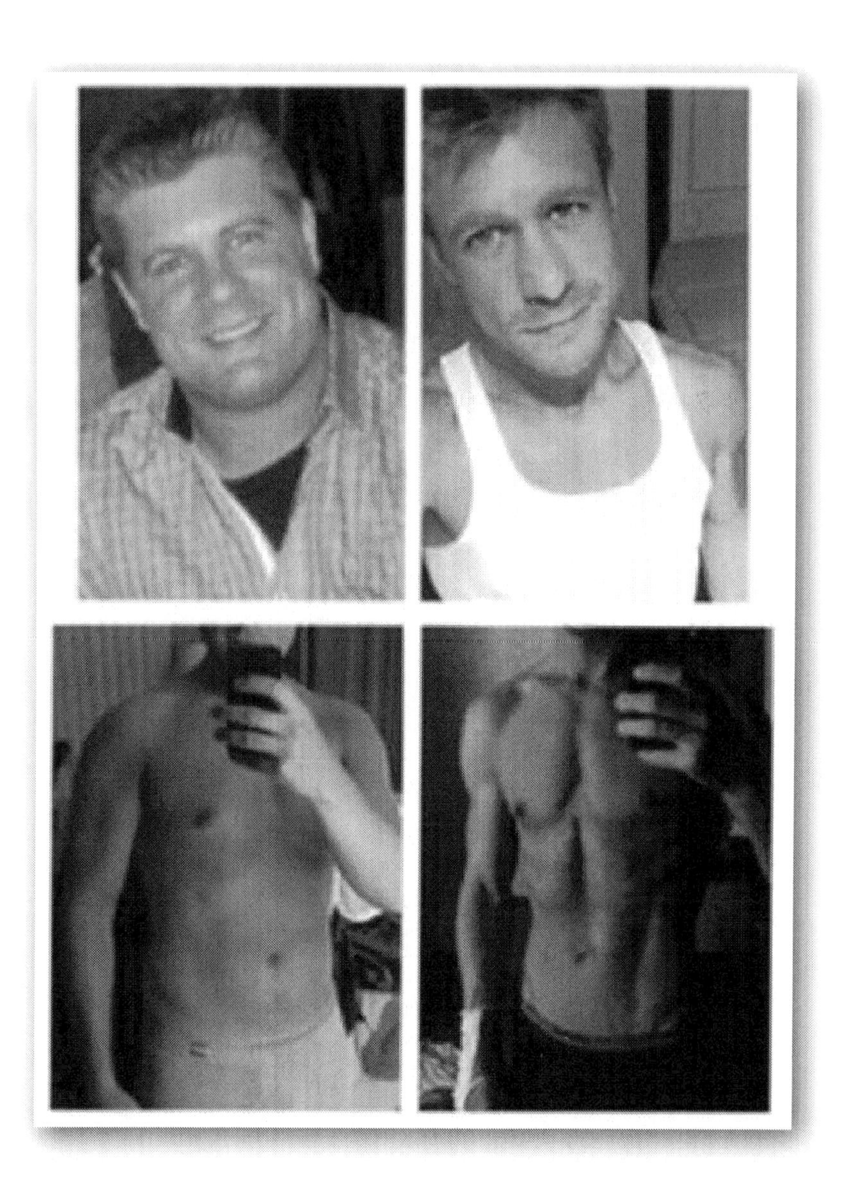

When I hit the 50 pounds lost mark, I got a tattoo as a reward. It's in Croatian and says, "Don't let your dreams be dreams," a quote from a Jack Johnson song that I've always really connected with and felt was relevant to my fitness achievement.

So I was able to add "being fit" to my list of all that was awesome in my life. But I still had an itch to leave Minnesota. Chase the ocean and beach of California for good. When I was at that work training in Colorado, I met a colleague, Tony, who currently lived in Huntington Beach, California. He and I got close those eight weeks. So in February, as I was just kicking off my fitness journey, I flew out to Huntington Beach to meet his family and take a little tour of the city.

Loved it. Very chill surfer city. Fun little downtown. Close to Los Angeles if I wanted to go to LA, but far enough away to mostly avoid the traffic and all the Hollywood/ celebrity blah blah. Tony's whole family was awesome... a group I would happily spend a lot of time with. Nice to know I'd have a couple good people I knew out there. Oh and the ocean. I had a crazy crush on the ocean.

So on a whim I said, "Screw it. I'm moving."

I found an amazing two-bedroom apartment with a large balcony one block from the ocean in early August. Packed up my stuff. My stepdad drove the moving truck out to California and I flew in.

I seriously had my life right where I wanted it. Unpacked all my stuff in California. Took advantage of the beach and the chance to be proud of taking my shirt off. Even lined up a first date that first weekend.

It's funny actually... I was doing some "manscaping" of my nether region in preparation for this date when I realized...

my left testicle is noticeably bigger than my right. Has it always been like that? Did I bump it while moving my stuff in or something? Meh.

I thought little of it and moved on. Fast-forward to three days later, and it had grown even more. I'm super stubborn when it comes to going to the doctor. But, I actually really like that area of my body... so I figured I'd book a urologist appointment ASAP. And then on Wednesday, September 3 ... 1 1/2 weeks after moving to California and starting my perfect life, I went to the urologist and by the end of the day everything in my life changed.

I got diagnosed with testicular cancer. The second I dropped my shorts for the urologist he was like, "We're going to do an ultrasound and get a second opinion from the radiologist in the hospital, but I can tell you now that you have testicular cancer."

I went home and made a dozen phone calls. Called my close friends, called my dad. My mom and stepdad were in France on vacation, so I figured I'd let them enjoy their vacation and I'd tell them two days later, on Friday, when they got home.

Everyone asked me, "How do you feel?" And truthfully, I wasn't scared at all. It was just more annoying. Like, ugh, I have to deal with this now. Great. I had just gotten into the best shape of my life. I had just moved to my dream area. It's never great timing to get a cancer diagnosis, but this was exceptionally bad timing.

At that time, we assumed the cancer was only in my testicle and that after a quick surgery, it would just be six weeks of recovery and I'd be back to good. Two days later, Friday, I was back with the urologist. He had the blood results. Bad blood results. Basically a guarantee that the cancer had spread from my testicle to somewhere else. After a CT scan we found that it was in my lymph nodes. A baseball-sized tumor was in my lymph nodes. This was where chemo was introduced. I'd need chemo now.

I was sitting in this appointment when my mom texted me saying she was back from France, but was still stuck on France time and was exhausted, and that she'd just talk to me tomorrow. She figured I just really wanted to hear about the trip. I replied like, "Hey, actually stay up. I'll call you really soon… kinda have something important to tell you."

The call to my mom and stepdad was like all the others. Shock. Asking what I need. The difference was, mom didn't take no for an answer when she said she was coming out to take care of me through this. She's a nurse. I'm her oldest baby. There was no convincing her otherwise. I said I needed a couple days of alone time but that she could get in the day before my first surgery. So that was that.

Anyway, I wanted to write this memoir to share the incredible support I had during my battle with cancer. From testicular surgery to chemo to lymph node surgery, I had such an incredible cast of characters making me smile, giving me hope, and praying for me. And nearly all of it came through social media… a place I least expected.

I'm so excited that you get to see my blog entries, my Instagram posts, and all the love I received from everyone who got to read them live. You'll see the funny and motivating comments in my blog entries, the random Instagram strangers wishing me luck from all over the world, sharing their stories of cancer, and telling me how inspired they are by my battle. Well, they inspired me! My friends, family, and total strangers gave me high hopes as I powered through this very, very tough time in my life. I hope this will inspire you too. To always fight. You're stronger than you know.

9-9-2014: Kickin' It With Mom

by ERIC GLYNN, Tuesday, September 9, 2014

Mom got here about 12 p.m. today. For as hard as I pushed her not to come, because it wasn't necessary, I'm very happy she's here. Gave her the quick tour of the apartment, showed her the 100 percent uncomfortable blow up mattress she's going to be rocking while she's here, and had an afternoon happy hour on my patio. We just got back from dinner where she got to meet the Borszcz family. So, I'm very happy she's here and all that.

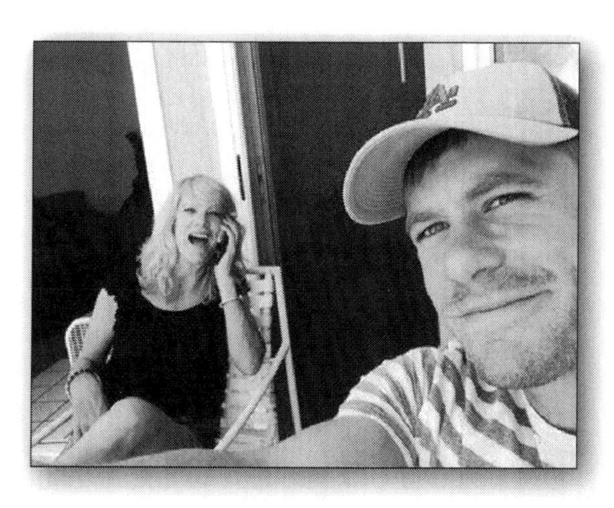

But what I really want to say... I truly, truly cannot explain how awesome these last 24 hours have been. I would never have imagined the number of Facebook messages, messages on this blog, texts, phone calls, emails... all with well-wishes and support. My senior year prom date called me to offer support yesterday, and I literally haven't heard her voice since I dropped her off at her house on prom night OVER 10 YEARS AGO. Former co-workers, Lakeville High School people, current super close friends, family... you've all been truly incredible. If I didn't think I'd hear from you, I heard from you. If I thought it would be a simple well wish, it was a phone call letting me know you'd be open to coming to Cali to hang, if I needed someone. A friend stopped by mom and Alan's last night with a bottle of whiskey and just sipped one down and chatted with them. Dozens of random people I have never met before reached out on Instagram and wished me the best on my surgery. For someone who hasn't always thought too highly of humanity at times, I seriously couldn't be more thankful for the love, in all forms, that I've received. I could keep going on this, but you get it. I'm blown away.

So, tomorrow. Mom and I have to get to the hospital at 3 p.m. to do some pre-surgery tests. Surgery starts at 5:30 p.m. Surgery shouldn't take too long, and then two hours of recovery after and we should be outta there between 8 and 9 p.m. tomorrow night, with me probably stumbling out of the hospital because:

A: I'll be crazy drugged up on pain meds *insert thumbs up emoji here*

B: I'll be re-calibrating my balance due to the fact that ONE OF MY BALLS WILL NOT BE IN MY BODY

ANYMORE AND WILL BE UNDER A MICROSCOPE BEING BIOPSIED.
So that's… *baller...* ;)

On Friday morning, we should have the results of the biopsy and we can take all the accumulated information, pass it along to USC, and schedule my first oncology visit to meet a couple of the doctors and come up with my chemo plan. Oh, chemo…

My urologist shared my info with a former patient of his who was a similar age and went through almost the exact same thing. That former patient, Peter, called me this morning and we talked for a little bit — all my questions were about the chemo. I asked for him to be blunt and straight up honest.

And it sounds truly awful.

He had to be out of work for five months. He couldn't walk to the end of the driveway to get his mail sometimes because he was feeling too weak. Lost all his hair and gained weight due to the steroids. Had to do many inpatient, week-long visits at USC for treatment. Got sick with a 106 degree temperature once… and really, even after stopping chemo after four months and recovering for one more before going back to work, he said he didn't have anywhere near the energy he had before chemo until a year after all of it started. So… ugh.

I wonder if I can manage this from Cali. Even if I end up staying right next door to USC… will I be able to get my own groceries, do my laundry… wipe my own ass? I won't know.

I really want to stay in California for treatment, heal up, and continue this new path I had JUST started two weeks ago, of Huntington Beach living. But I also won't be stubborn about throwing up the white flag and saying, "Dammit, I need to go back to Minnesota for this."

Question for the group: It sounds like I can collect social security or disability pay or some crap during my chemo with a doctor's note and reaching out to the state.

Does anyone know much about any of that? Does anyone also know if there's a law or rules that protect me from getting terminated from my company if I have documentation from my oncologist saying I literally cannot work for 4-5 months or however long chemo will last? Like, is illness in the same ballpark as pregnancy, as far as being legally protected and stuff? Any basic information or contact names of people who would be willing to give me an overview would be awesome. Chatting with my company's HR department tomorrow to review options there.

To finish up, I'm in good spirits, guys. My chemo talk with that former patient was scary and it truly sounds AWFUL, AWFUL, AWFUL, but I want to get it started as soon as I can after surgery and have it just be done as soon as possible. Again, I truly can't tell you how much the random acts of service, messages, and well-wishes have meant to me and the family over the last day. You all are amazing. I look forward to the day that I'm the "former patient" and I can freak out some cancer newbie with the blunt honesty about chemo, but let him know that it's curable, and you come out all good on the other side. I can't wait to be a success story.

I'll say "hey" as early as I am able after my surgery tomorrow night.

Favorite Comments

Eric - you have an AMAZING attitude and with that you will come out ahead!! I hope surgery goes well!
—Nicole Dixon, September 10, 2014

Nobody ever needed two balls anyway.
—Karen Feldman, September 10, 2014

Wow, you are a courageous young man that hasn't lost your sense of humor. (I think you get that from your mother). Move on forward and get this experience behind you. Keep the faith and your sense of humor and all will be well.
—Pam McDonald, September 10, 2014

Instagram 9-10-14 @eric_t_glynn

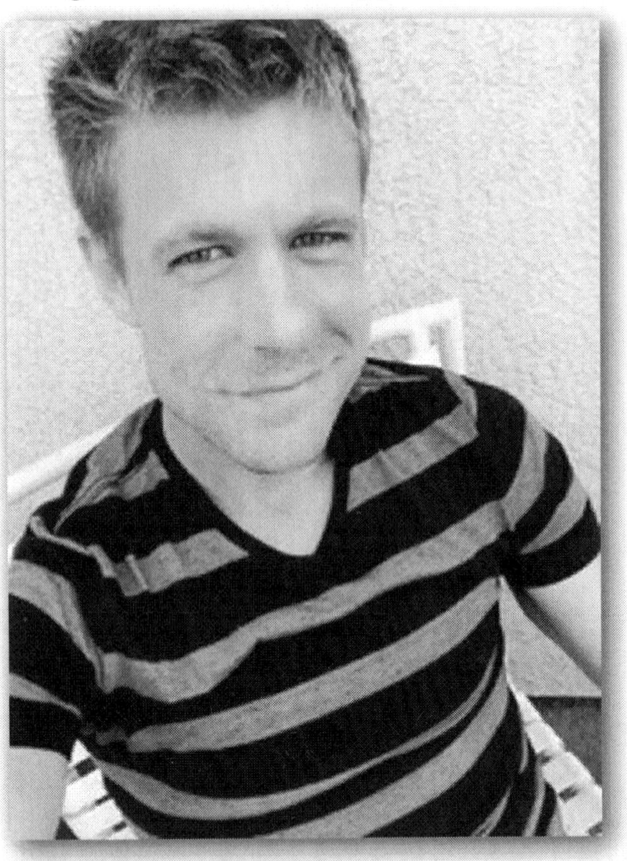

I have some rough news, all. I'm having major surgery on Wednesday that will keep me bed ridden and unable to lift and do cardio for 4-6 weeks. So while my fitness journey is on hold, I hope to start so many more on theirs! Reach out through Direct Message with questions, before/after pics...I wanna be a part of your journey while mine is on pause! I hope to heal up fast and get back to posting my lovely douchy-selfies-of-the-day again real soon :) -Eric #douchyselfieoftheday #starttoday #fitness #workout #gym #weightlifting #fitfam #weightloss #selfie #cali #california #socal #westcoast #huntingtonbeach #hb #ca #la #losangeles #DMme

Favorite Comments

@thu***

Sending love and healing!!

@pun***

You're so sweet to want to help others whilst resting up yourself. If you want a chat to keep you occupied just drop me a message.

@gin***

Your eyes say there are more things to come. Bigger, better things.

@eric_t_glynn

@gin***** aw I really like that comment about the eyes. I think you're right about that ;)

@cat***

You are seriously bloody beautiful! And my God, I've never seen anyone project so much positivity to the world. You seriously are an inspiration! Looking forward to seeing you come through this. Mind over matter is half the battle! PS, did I mention you are seriously beautiful? Haha xx

@jad***

My thoughts and prayers are with you... one of my best friends was just diagnosed last week :/

9-11-2014: Um, Ouch...

by ERIC GLYNN, Thursday, September 11, 2014

I'm alive. The operation went perfectly yesterday. But holy mother eff it hurts. After I came to from the anesthesia in the hospital I was shaking uncontrollably from the pain, so the awesome nurse kept pumping drugs and drugs and drugs into the IV for me. Each dose calmed the shaking and made my pain number go from like 8 to 7 to 6 to 5 to 4... and then I drank a little water, the first time I'd had something to eat or drink in 13 hours. I asked if they had any whiskey, pointing out the fact that liquor is sterile... but it was a poorly received question.

Got wheeled to mom, and my last task was to stand up and prove I could pee on my own before I got to leave. The former cancer patient I talked to yesterday said that he had to try like a half-a-dozen times before it worked, and I kinda chuckled at him about that. Cut to last night, where I'm standing over the can, wondering why in the hell I can't take a leak. I'm approaching a "too much information" zone here, but I tried standing, sitting, standing, sitting, running water... aaaand then after about five minutes, I almost passed out due to the pain. Soooooo... the very patient nurse walked me back to my bed with all my urine still in my bladder and a fussy look on my face. Couple minutes later I marched back into that damn bathroom, pissed like a champ, and we rolled out of there.

Then we went to CVS to get drugs, and there was a big crap show around them needing to call my doctor to confirm I was legitimately allowed to get the pain meds. So we had to call my doctor, at like midnight, for him to authorize it. Mom was an angry, protective mama bird at this point and emotionally scarred the pharmacist, I think. Nah, she wasn't super mean, but we had both just had it for the day.

Anyway, got me home, I made a couple quick calls and went to bed. Slept pretty deep for an hour at a time, but obviously woke up a bunch due to the ouchiness. Mom said that I had to call out to her anytime I needed to get up at night to use the bathroom. She's gonna be grumpy when she reads this, but I got up like four or five times during the night to use the bathroom without her help. Sorry Mudder!! :D :D :D :D :D

So today's schedule is as follows:

8 a.m.-10 p.m.: Lay on my couch

Mom's schedule is as follows:

8:00 a.m.: Get Eric an energy drink
8:30 a.m.: Get Eric an energy drink
9:00 a.m.: Get Eric an energy drink... etc...

Favorite Comments

dancing with you buddy! Mama FOSS!
—Chris Foss, September 12, 2014

In the land of the blind the man with one eye is king and in the land of the skunk the man with half a nose is king. I'm not sure what land it would be but I think having one ball makes you a king somewhere.
—Justin McMartin, September 11, 2014

Mama Michelle - I have always loved your spunk. That pharmacist went home with a "hell of a night" story – proud of you, girl! Eric - don't do anything to bring that side of your mom out... like being too strong in the middle of the night by yourself. John and I have been lifting you both, the doctors, nurses and your extended family up in prayer. We will continue and continue. Thank you for the updates - your strength is admirable!!! Much love!!
—Kristin Ritter, September 11, 2014

Glad you're back home friend! Way to show that bladder you're the boss. Give your mother a hug and remember to say your prayers. S'later.
—Anthony Giorgi, September 11, 2014

Remember, if you shake more than three times, you're just playing with it.
—David Slifka, September 11, 2014

Glad you're on the mend! Way to go potty on the potty! ;) Continued prayers of healing and comfort for you and prayers of patience and endurance for your mom!
—Sarah Johnson, September 11, 2014

Instagram 9-12-2014 @eric_t_glynn

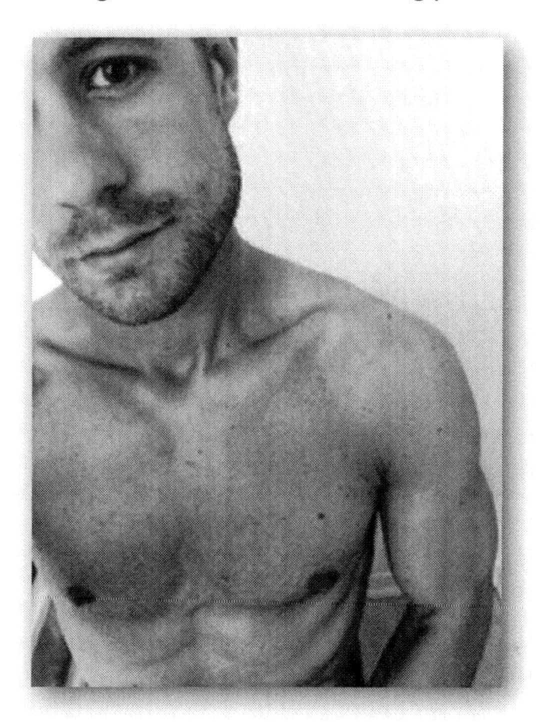

So I want to share some more about my health. Surgery was successful yesterday. It was surgery to remove cancer that I was diagnosed with last Wednesday. Unfortunately the cancer has spread and I'm looking at 4-5 months of chemo. From January 1 to today I've completely changed my nutrition, cardio and lifting, losing 60 pounds and getting into the best shape of my life, but that's nothing compared to the challenge I'm about to face. I will lose my hair, become frail. Be sick every day. But dammit, I'm going to come out the other side stronger inside and out. I have a blog I'm keeping about my journey, feel free to read it and leave comments, or DM me here. I'm open to answering questions about fitness or hear stories or questions about cancer here. I created this to help people, and I want to continue doing so even if my fitness journey has absolutely slammed to a halt and a chemo/cancer journey has begun. #douchyselfieoftheday #starttoday #fitness #workout #gym #weightlifting #cancer #chemo #support

Favorite Comments

@ani***

:'(I know you can pull through, you've conquered one journey and you can conquer this one too. Stay strong!

@dan***

Good luck!!! Good juju your way!!! I'm so inspired by your journey! Don't let this hiccup stop you!

@x_c***

Wow, my regards are with you. If you pulled off all the weight you can pull this cancer off. Keep going, be strong and our prayers are with you!!!

@her***

Be strong! Be positive! Have lots of faith, God is with you. I will have you in my thoughts and prayers sending the best energy and thoughts. Wish you the best and lots of success. Lots of hugs and support from this end to you, buddy. Wish you the best outcome of this, you are a warrior. Keep your head up.

@hea***

Stay strong and keep a positive attitude! Over the past year I have had several surgeries to have cancerous cells removed. I never had to go through chemo, but it was always a struggle being in and out of recovery. You've got this!

@not***

Losing weight was like a warm up. You did that and now you can beat cancer! Wish you the best.

@eric_t_glynn

Thank each and every one of you so much. The struggle has already begun, but I can't stop won't stop. You'll see...

@all***

#livestrong my mom just went through chemo, it's a bitch but you can kick cancer's ass just like she did!

@rob***

Wow, was being a bit superficial and just looking at your pics. Now I'm reading the content. Seems like someone who has lost that much weight out of pure discipline, is definitely a fighter. Looks like you've got a healthy mind, now keep on fighting and you'll have a healthy body soon enough!

9-13-2014: Preliminary Biopsy Results

by ERIC GLYNN, Saturday, September 13, 2014

Wassup my cancer army? I know I sound like a broken record, but all the support has been incredible. Mom and I have gotten a kick out of all the comments here, Facebook stuff, texts, emails and calls. I had no, no, no idea I'd have the support group that I do, and I can't even scratch the surface on how amazing it all is. To have people I don't know reach out and say, "I know you don't know me, but ____ told me about what you're going through and I just want you to know that I'm thinking about you,"... is just crazy to me.

Three days after surgery and the pain is much better. I can sleep on my side like I like to, and can get up, sit down, do everything I have to, without help. I'm proud to announce that I've been independent enough to where my mom hasn't had to see or help me with my penis once! We're both relieved...

A few updates: My doc called me yesterday with some preliminary results on the cancer they pulled. Apparently, I'm sitting at Stage 2 Testicular Cancer, with one of the two cancers they found being Embryonal Carcinoma. This is a very aggressive cancer that hauls ass and spreads around the body like a son of a bitch (so it makes sense that it's already all over my lymph nodes). We're going to need to be very proactive and quick to jump start chemo before it gets bored with the organs it's already chillin' in and chooses to continue on its destructive path and latch on elsewhere.

So we'll have the final biopsy report first thing Monday. We have my first oncology visit scheduled for Tuesday at 2:30 p.m. at USC. We will walk out of there with a plan for chemo, which, according to my doctor, will almost certainly be months of a repeating pattern of going into the hospital and being inpatient for a full week, while they inject me with the chemo, and then two weeks of resting at home before going back in for more.

In dealing with all the HR stuff at work, I can be placed on short-term and then long-term disability, to where I will collect 60 percent of my base, up to two years and three months, with doctor's notes. They don't take any commissions I'd make as a salesman into account. So with that, there's no way I can afford the apartment and Huntington Beach living, so I will need to leave the apartment I just moved into 2 1/2 weeks ago. I'm going to the property management building Monday morning and will play the cancer card to see if I can just get out of my year lease with no penalties. Hopefully someone in there has a soul and will let that happen. I've already paid for September rent, so I'll have until the end of the month to get all my stuff outta here. My plan is to put all the big stuff into storage out here, because the second I'm all cleaned up, my goal is to be back here, as Huntington Beach is amazing and there are such good people here.

So my last real decision is where to do chemo. I love Cali so much, and my spirits would be the highest here, so the USC option looks very attractive. We have a family friend with an apartment 20 minutes from USC that I could stay in, free of charge. The big issue is the support and help I'll need while I'm doing chemo. In reading the former cancer patient, Peter's CaringBridge journal of his time going through this exact same chemo three years ago, it sounds like I will be just worthless during chemo. There were multiple times where issues arose at home with fevers and things to where he had to be admitted to the hospital during his off weeks.

So, I wonder if it would be at all possible to handle that on my own out here.

I could get my groceries delivered, I could have a cleaning service do my laundry and tidy up the apartment... it's just the 3 a.m., 106 degree fevers and medical emergencies that I sit and think, can I handle this? These are the questions that we'll be bringing to USC, and if they straight up say, "No way man," my only real option would be to head back to Minnesota for treatment at either Mayo Clinic or Minnesota Oncology in Minneapolis.

I have an aunt and uncle living in Rochester, Minnesota, who actually work for Mayo Clinic, who could help out and I'd hope to be in Lakeville with mom and Alan or in Blaine with dad and Mary and the kids during my off weeks, if I'm up for the driving and all that. It would be nice to have the familiarity of "home" during those rest weeks. My biggest concern is that there's good wifi in the locations I'll be living, as I plan to play the crap out of video games online the whole time! I'll also probably watch literally everything that Netflix has to offer.

It appears, though, that once chemo kicks up, I'll be freaking exhausted and I may not have much energy. Mom will be able to post journals on my behalf to keep everyone updated.

I'll also say it now, while I have a clear mind... don't be offended if I'm in rough shape a ton of the time and can't take visitors when the chemo is pulsing through me. I'll be super honest about whether it's a good day or not, and may have to turn away people if I'm just death-bedding it.

I'll close with another motivation to crush cancer. I have a buddy in San Francisco who is about to send me some Ferrari hats. Sounds like after my first week of chemo and two weeks of home, my hair will be gone. I'll be wearing the hats to the sessions, and he said that the day cancer is gone, he's picking me up in his Ferrari and we're going to joyride up Pacific Coast Highway in Cali and just soak it all in. If I could drive a stick I'd implore him to let me drive, but I'll be cool in the passenger seat gunning it 100 mph up the Cali coast. :)

Favorite Comments

Eric - I knew you more as a little boy and to hear you "talk" now as a young man just makes me feel as proud as your mom probably feels! You are being incredibly strong and your humor is helping the rest of us be strong, too! Because you get away with "potty mouth" I feel like I can, too. So with that... I have been praying at the craziest of moments for you - I'm a teacher and whenever I see one of the boys I work with holding his penis = prayer time for Eric! You wouldn't believe how many times boys do that! Well, maybe you would believe it - you're a boy :) Anyway, you have lots and lots of prayers coming your way. Give your mom a GIANT hug from me. Thank you for the updates (from you AND Eric's mom) - Love and blessings, Kristin

—Kristin Ritter, September 13, 2014

I have some baseball hats. All yours if you want them. You are stronger than you even know right now. And you will find even more strength as you go. Straight ahead Eric. You have our prayers.
—Mark Foss, September 13, 2014

Okay, let's be honest, the most significant factor in your decision is sunset picture opportunities.
—Justin McMartin, September 13, 2014

You're my hero. Keep on keeping on with that Ball Bunyan attitude and you'll destroy this cancer. No question about it. It sounds as though you have an army behind you that's ready to help you fight this war. Anytime you need me to "awkward trout" the hell out of you, let me know!
—Katie Laschinger, September 13, 2014

Awww, Eric you are so awesome and so inspiring!! If anyone can beat this you WILL. We will be sad to see you go, but we know it may be the best option and it'll be temporary, for you will soon enough be enjoying the HB sunshine again and we will be here to celebrate with you!! In the meantime, we're here for you and your mom for WHATEVER you need. Oh, and I'm bringing you some Nutella today...
—Teresa Borszcz, September 13, 2014

9-15-2014: Los Angeles

by ERIC GLYNN, Monday, September 15, 2014

So this morning, mom and I drove up to Los Angeles to meet with the family who would let me stay at their apartment during chemo, should I opt for treatment at USC. The place is very nice, in an incredibly cool area. There is a concierge who I can call for food delivery, cleaning service, etc. So all that stuff would be taken care of. The apartment is a great 2 bedroom, 2 1/2 bath, two-story place, fully furnished, two balconies, with almost literally everything I need. I'd just have to pack up some clothes, a couple video game systems and drive Ruby, my Mercedes Benz, on up to it. I'd put everything else into storage in Huntington Beach so it'll be right there when I return in glorious victory.

The couple who owns the place is incredible. I'd get to stay for free and have all utilities covered. Very nice, genuine people who want to help. This is all changing my outlook on people. Didn't like too many people all that much going in, but the outreach has been insane. How many times have I said that? Enough, I bet.

So tomorrow at 2 p.m. is my first appointment with the oncologists. They have all my results and we will walk out of there with their proposed chemo plan. After tomorrow's visit, everything will move super fast. I'll have to pack up and move out of my Huntington Beach apartment and hopefully get out of that lease with a property management visit. I plan to bring my big blue-green puppy eyes and play the cancer card for help. Oh and bring a doctor's note. I'll have to decide on whether USC is the spot for me or if I need second and third opinions in Minnesota. I have to line up my disability and inform work of everything. After I can check all that GARBAGE off my list, I can just focus on getting healthy.

So yeah, tomorrow will be a big, informative day. If the cancer will allow me a couple weeks to tackle all that BS in the above paragraph before I start chemo, that would be great. But they may say, "Hey, if you have time right now, let's pump a little ooze into you today and get things started because seriously, your cancer is a jackass and is making its next move." I gotta be ready for that too.

I'm sure a big ole post will show up in your inbox tomorrow when we get all the facts.

I'll close with the most important news of all over the last two days. The Borszcz family came over yesterday for mom's world famous "Sloppy Joes," and they brought Nutella with them. It was the first time I ever tried Nutella. And OMG. Nutella, you guys. I've already gained 250 lbs and its Nutella's fault. I'm gonna ask the oncologists if they can mix the chemo drugs with some Nutella before they shoot it in my veins, because it seriously can only help...

Favorite Comments

Hey Eric I know today is a major day!! The only thing you can control is your attitude and you have an awesome one! Love is all around you!!
—Lisa Yetzer, September 16, 2014

All your Indy peeps have been keeping you in their prayers… including our little guys! Btw, should you be making us all laugh with these posts? Shouldn't it be the other way around… I am thinking a book deal might be in your future!
—Leah Hobbs, September 16, 2014

9-16-2014: Treatment Plan Is SET

by ERIC GLYNN, Tuesday, September 16, 2014

This is going to be a long post.

Mom and I went to my oncology appointment today. We got to meet my wonderful oncology doc, Dr. Tanya Dorff, and she walked us through the chemo plan. This is going to be a long, long journey. I'm gonna put all the chemo medical jargon and crap in here for those who are scientific or have had people they know go through chemo. Everyone else will be like, "Wtffffff are you talking about??????" Don't worry, you're with the 99.99 percent of the population on that one.

Here's my path:

—Nine weeks of chemo to start. The chemo will be in three cycles of three weeks. Each cycle is one week of chemo, Monday through Friday, 8 a.m. to 5 p.m. The second and third weeks of chemo are considered "rest" weeks, where I'll only go in for chemo on Tuesdays for one hour. The first week I'll get the Bleomycin and Etoposide treatments all five days, along with the Cisplatin treatment on the Tuesday of that week. On my two "rest" weeks, the Tuesday treatment will be the Cisplatin. So, three cycles of three weeks. At the end of the nine weeks, they'll look at my numbers and see if all is in line, or if we need to do an additional three-week cycle. So, in total, chemo will be between nine and 12 weeks.

—After chemo is complete, I will have a three to four week total rest period to get all the chemo out of there.

—Because the tumor in my lymph nodes is so large, there's no way chemo will completely get rid of it. It will just shrink it enough to where they can operate on it. So after my three to four weeks of rest, I will have surgery to remove the remaining tumor. The slice will be straight down my stomach from my chest bone to my belly button. Recovery from the surgery is 12 weeks or three months.

SO, including chemo, rest, surgery and surgery recovery, we're looking at 25 to 28 weeks. A. Half. A. Year! I will be out of work for that full period.

Anyway, after meeting with these folks at USC, I've decided I'm doing chemo and surgery here in California. I will be staying at the apartment in Glendale, California, which is 20 minutes from USC.

This is not a popular decision to family and many friends, but this is best for Eric. Truly. My spirits will be highest in California. I love my doctors and the facility already. The decision is made.

So, chemo starts Monday. As in six days from now, Monday. Between now and then I need to: let work know about all this, work with UNUM to get on disability, work with my property management company to get out of my Huntington Beach lease, get a Uhaul lined up to pick up the stuff from my

Huntington Beach apartment, which means packing up everything and planning and sorting what I'll need during all of this in LA, schedule moving people to pack my stuff into the Uhaul and then drop off into a storage facility in Huntington Beach, which I also need to schedule and book. This will all be happening Wednesday through Friday this week. On Saturday or Sunday I will be moving into the LA apartment for good and then Monday it all starts.

So between right now and the weekend, I'm going to be a ghost. Don't get all fussy with me if I don't reply to texts, emails and calls over the next couple days, cuz I'll soooorrrt-taaaa have my hands full. :) I'll keep everyone posted here as best I can, but these next couple days will be nuts. It will feel so good when this is all lined up, I'm all checked into LA, and I can just focus on healing up.

I feel like there's more I should be saying right now, but my brain is everywhere else. So off I go.

Ah, DAMMIT, I forgot to ask the oncologists if there's a chance I'll get a superpower from the chemicals in the chemo. I'll take the power of flight or invisibility... or even the ability to not be as directionally challenged as I am. Is that too much to ask??

Favorite Comments

Is baldness considered a superpower? Because maybe you could blind people with your soon-to-be shiny head. Or maybe your power could be to bike really fast because I'm sure the aerodynamics of one testicle is how Lance Armstrong won all those races.

—Scott Deeney, September 17, 2014

ENDS WITH A ZINGER!!!! That's some high school speech team ish right there.
—Mike Glynn, September 17, 2014

I'm sure your unemployment will be offset now that you won't have to buy two types of hair gel. Keep strong homey.
—David Slifka, September 17, 2014

Instagram 9-17-14 @eric_t_glynn

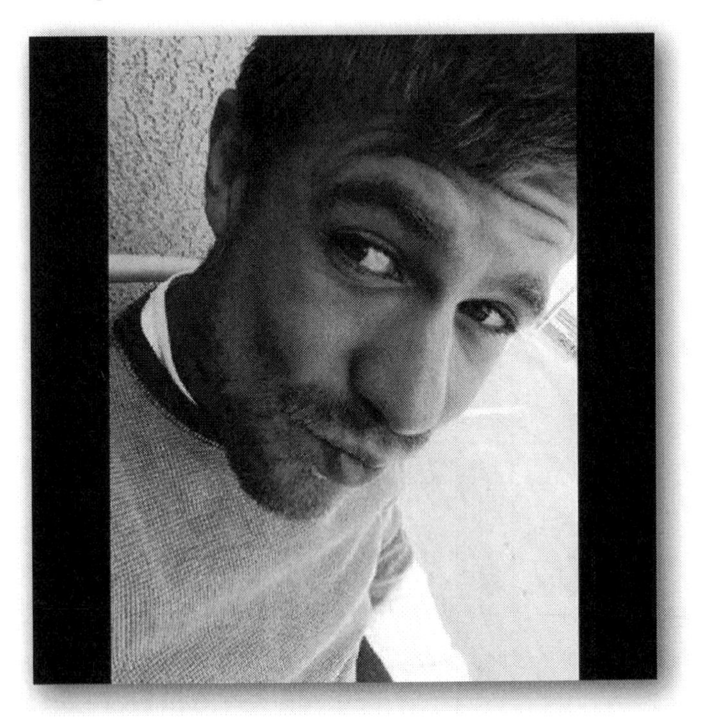

This will be my last pic with hair. Chemo starts Monday. I'm about to embark on a 25-week journey of chemo and surgery to get rid of my cancer. My next pic will be me in my chemo. I'll be bald and not look great at all. I'm going to show you what chemo does, how it rocks you, so that when I'm on the other side you can see how strong you can (and I am going to) come back from it, you'll see what is possible. The Direct Messages and comments with well wishes and hopes and prayers have been incredible. I will always be checking IG through this for cancer support, fitness questions, etc. The support of you total strangers is truly amazing. I will dominate this and come out stronger on the other side. #douchyselfieoftheday #starttoday #fitness #workout #gym #weightlifting #fitfam #weightloss #selfie #cali #california #socal #westcoast #huntingtonbeach #hb #ca #la #losangeles #DMme #cancer #chemo #support

Favorite Comments

@my_*****

@my_*****

You'll kick cancer in the teeth and dominate! I have faith in you, sweetheart.

@nee***

Wishing you strength while going through chemo. You clearly have a positive attitude, which will only help you. Positive thoughts and prayers your way.

@drj***

May you conquer this with strength, love and determination. Find hope and comfort in others around you, friend or stranger. People care a lot more than we think. :) God bless.

@bri***

You are so incredibly strong, beyond words. You have shown your determination through your fitness journey and I have no doubt that you will come back stronger than every before. All the best, love all the way from NZ <3

@mis***

I don't know you but besides being handsome you look like a really strong individual. My brother went through cancer and I just want to tell you to never stop fighting and being optimistic. It makes a difference. God bless you, I'm sure you will be okay.

@cra***

Your determination is inspiring! This has made me realize my "problems" are not that bad. Here I am bitching and moaning about being fat and tired, both of which are a) not that bad and b) totally fixable :) Best of luck to you!

@nic***

Thanks for the like. I was touched by your story and just want to send positive vibes. Remember that "God gives His hardest battles to His strongest warriors." Hang in there pal!

@mer***

Hi!! Wow, you're a fighter. I adore you, I wish you the best. I'm gonna pray for you and always remember that you have a friend that's always going to be supporting you from Mexico. Kisses and hugs!!

@nen***

Through your posts I gather you have a beautiful spirit! I'm sure your words are encouraging to others traveling a similar path :) Stay strong and beautiful, no struggle is in vain! <3

9-18-2014: Never A Dull Day

by ERIC GLYNN, Thursday, September 18, 2014

So we thought Wednesday would be a chill day. Get the packing going, do some administrative stuff. Aaaaand then we talked to my oncologist. My blood results from Tuesday came back. Again, I dunno the science and biology, but when comparing my blood numbers from a week ago to Tuesday's, things have gotten far worse. One of the levels has doubled. Another has jumped up a large amount. My official full-recovery-o'meter went from "good" to "intermediate." Basically they told me that it's super important that we start everything as soon as possible, but that we can still wait for our originally planned Monday start date. There are also some special chemo drugs that could be really, really helpful for me that I'd qualify for since I'm in the intermediate stage, but it's a bit of a lotto chance that I'd be administered them as I've been added to a study where some of the patients will receive them and some won't. Even if I don't get those, I still have a kick ass chemo plan set up and am ready to rock for Monday.

This does mean, however, that instead of three cycles of three weeks of chemo, that we will HAVE to do four cycles of three weeks of chemo. No way around that. This bumps my chemo, surgery and recovery time to 28 weeks, minimum. So we're looking at mid-April to be fully functional after the final surgery, and that's when I could begin a job search as a cancer-clear, surgery recovered dude. Mid-April. That's right around the corner, right?

Anyway, so they let us know that because it will be four cycles of three weeks of chemo, my semen is probably going to get fried and suggested I hit up a sperm bank. So… I did that yesterday. I'll hold back on most of the details. Lets just say there was a TV with a DVD ready to go when I got in the ole, um, "action room," and then "stuff" happened. So I dunno what you were doing at 1:30 p.m. yesterday, but I was…

Moving on. So that was tough to hear that things are getting lamer inside my dumb body, but there's some good news too. In looking over my upcoming budget for the seven-plus months of cancer killing, and factoring in the disability pay that I'll fortunately get to take in, the numbers are enough in my favor that I will be able to hold onto my Huntington Beach apartment. So the stress of packing up EVERYTHING, trying to get out of my lease, renting a Uhaul and movers, renting a storage shed, and taking all my stuff there, is GONE. I can't describe how many stressors this kills for me over the next couple days. Mom and I have been able to focus on getting all my appointments lined up and I'll just have to pack what I need to bring up to LA, which won't be a lot. Also, when mom drives me effing crazy or vice versa, we have a place for one of us to disappear to for the weekend, or a place for one of us to go if/when she or I have guests in to visit. So, so fortunate that things have lined up this way.

Finally, a huge, huge "Thank you" for everything. Someone sent me a ton of food, tea, nausea stuff. I've gotten many cards.

A bouquet of chocolate was left at my apartment. You all are too much. I'm sorry I don't have the time to thank you all individually, but hopefully all the senders are able to see this. You all are amazing. And you're amazing.

Also, you're amazing.

Favorite Comments

So, I never thought I'd see the day that I would tell my son to go masturbate and to do his best. And then pray that it goes well. :)
This has been an odd day.
Love, Mom
—Eric's mom, September 19, 2014

YOU and YOU are amazing!! Here we all sit in the comfort of our homes reading and praying for you - we have it easy! Thank you so very much for the updates - each of you have an incredible amount of emotional and physical strength. I've decided that when I grow up, I want to be as crazy funny and tell it like it is as each of you! Big favor - If you'd be willing to share what you specifically need to make each moment a teeny bit easier, I (and I'm sure many others) would love to help – gas cards for the traveling, food cravings, drink cravings, any simple pleasure that we can provide, please please, please let us know. Have to end this with another thank you to Eric. Eric, I am thrilled that you are going to make your mom go to church this Sunday. :) Hold her hand and reassure her that you feel so lucky to go on such a great date with such a great woman! Love and huge prayers to you, both of you.
—Kristin Ritter, September 19, 2014

Sorry to hear about the recent results man, bummer to hear things take a turn. Hopefully they get you in on the trial, sounds like you're in good hands either way though. Also, thanks for not calling me to "lend a hand" at the ole spank bank, that may have been pushing the friendship a bit too far. Glad they had your niche preferences in stock, didn't think they could commit that stuff to DVD.

Good luck getting everything squared away prior to Monday, that's awesome you'll get to keep the Huntington Beach place through it. One less hassle is always good.
—Will Meacham, September 19, 2014

Hi Eric… I'm a coworker of your moms… thinking of you and hoping for the best. Gotta say I love your attitude and how positive you are… keep it up, that's the best medicine and you WILL kick cancer in the butt!!
—Melissa Siebenaler, September 19, 2014

TMI, but it's good our babies still have a chance at cousins some day. It sounds like you will be well enough just in time to come make an embarrassing best man speech... which I suppose I'm looking forward to :)
—Kristy Maguire, September 19, 2014

I wish I was doing that 1:30 yesterday.
—Bill Yetzer, September 19, 2014

You have such a great attitude and you are an amazing guy, Eric. Your journal entries always make me laugh, it should be the other way around! April... yeah that's really soon. Now I have 2 things to look forward to in April: hearing you are 100% cancer free and Game of Thrones Season 5! I'll say that I'm more excited about you being cancer free, and that's saying A LOT! :)
—Kelly Bundy, September 19, 2014

9-21-2014: Chemo Starts Tomorrow

by ERIC GLYNN, Sunday, September 21, 2014

We are all settled into LA. Chemo starts tomorrow and at 8 a.m. I get my port put in. It's a one-hour surgery. It's a plastic device they insert in my chest that connects to my heart or my veins or something where they'll draw blood from and pump the happy chemo drugs into from here on out. It'll be underneath the skin and will remain inside my chest until the cancer is clear. I think it's gonna look exactly like Ironman's chest thing… at least I'll ask if they have one of those for me. Either way, I'm walking into the hospital in an Ironman suit tomorrow. So… egg on my face if all they have are normal ports.

So after that we'll be waiting a bit and then I'll have my first chemo session. Should be somewhere around five hours as only two of the three chemo drugs will be pumped into me tomorrow. I believe the order is fluids, steroids, Chemo 1, Chemo 2.

So that should be great.

I'll be bringing my iPad, iPhone and iMac with me. So basically, it's gonna be Apple and I chillin' for a while. I won't know if I'm getting the regular drugs or the experimental ones until tomorrow morning sometime. Either way, I'm just ready to get started.

I can noticeably feel the tumor in my side when I move. It was 9cm by 5cm two weeks ago. It's grown for sure. Kinda gross. But yeah, I can feel it.

10 days later, and I'm 100 times better on my first surgery recoup. I still can't do cardio for three more weeks or any heavy lifting for five. I hope I'm at least sort of up for some working out during the rest weeks, or I'm going to go crazy. I do kind of have a badass master bedroom setup though, with a king-sized bed, large bathroom with a mini-jacuzzi, a TV with my Playstation 3 and Xbox One hooked up, and mom's a bell ring away from delivering me cookies and Redbull.

"Ma! The meatloaf!"

So again, this week is five days of chemo, followed by two rest weeks... aka my first cycle of four.

This area is absolutely amazing. Mom is very excited to explore the shops and restaurants. I know I will not be excited to explore anything outside my apartment as I'll be death-bedding it most of the time. If I could afford $4k-a-month, there are lovely apartments close by that would be fun to live in after this. Alas, I can't afford $4k-a-month.

During this downtime I'm going to think about possible career changes. Something in nutrition perhaps... maybe even with cancer. Like how you should eat and how far you can push yourself, cardio and weight-lifting wise, while you're going through chemo. Some type of coach like that, maybe in the LA-area. Could be cool. I'm thinking of starting a blog on how I lost all my weight and stuff while I lay in bed getting green stuff shot in my veins. I dunno, throwing all this stuff around and I'll see what comes out the other side.

There's a Fantastic Sams right by this apartment, so we're planning to get me a buzz cut this upcoming weekend, as my hair should start falling out next week. :/ ... I guess a buzz cut is better than CLUMPS OF HAIR falling out in bed and in the shower. I mean, unless you guys wanna see a clump-of-hair selfie? Maybe I can somehow form it into a "duckface?" I wouldn't put it past me...

I'll write another one of these as I'm getting my first treatment because that should be weird/interesting.

Favorite Comments

Hey Eric - I've always liked your style. There is nothing you can't beat. GO get it my friend. You've got this. And when you feel like you don't - looks like you have an amazing support system of friends and family all around you. Virtual hugs, Lil
—Lillian Malkin, September 23, 2014

Been thinking about you all day little buddy. You've got such a great spirit & attitude. Praying for that to continue. But if by chance you have moments of frustration or anger and you feel like you need to punch something... I volunteer Uncle Paul!
—Amy Glynn, September 22, 2014

I love the "fight" in you, Eric! You are going to beat this cancer and will have a "better" future because of what you're going through. Read "Romans 8:28" - it helps me keep things in perspective during difficult times. You and your mom continue to be in my prayers!
—Cathy Deeney, September 22, 2014

Good luck today!! I will be thinking of you in an Ironman suit all morning :) Thanks for that image. ;) You will ROCK it!
—Anne Simon, September 22, 2014

Hi Eric, I have never met anyone who has made their treatment sound quite so entertaining. I feel guilty for chuckling when you are going through such a tough time. I love you and continue to lift you up each day to God! Keep up the great spirit! Lots of love, Mary
—Mary Yetzer, September 21, 2014

Eric - tomorrow is a big day. While the chemo drips in, let your mind and body fight the cancer too. Visualize the fight going on. The cancer cells getting samurai attacked by the chemo... kind of like, I suspect, when you were a kid and wore a cape and something like Scooby-doo (or Turtles) undies and fought the bad guys with pretend swords... and LOUD verbal sword-rending sounds. In your mind, let it rip again… but this time fighting for real... and know our prayers are giving you lots of ammunition and higher fighting skills for this job. Will be praying tomorrow for you and mom... glad you took time to enjoy life and each other this weekend... weekends are for playing anyways, right?
—Roxy McGraw, September 21, 2014

Hi -Eric and Michelle (I work with your mom), you are both being amazing. Whether you believe in divine intervention or not, your humor and positive attitude are a winning combination. Though the medical stuff is your focus, it is so good to hear that you are getting out and doing something else to divert your attention a little. We miss your mom's sunshiney personality at work but know you are benefitting from it, even if you aren't always so sure... and this is the one time you will be glad to have a nurse in your family… it will make all the difference. I and everyone I know, are rooting for you both and if there is anything I/we can do from this end, please feel free. All the best moving forward.
—Jayne Marshall, September 21, 2014

Bring out the gloves, let the fight begin!!!! Time to knock this cancer on its ass. ;) Thinking of you and praying for peace, strength and patience as you move forward tomorrow. You got this one Eric!!!!! Loves!
—Cindy Weber, September 21, 2014

9-22-2014: Day One Of Chemo

by ERIC GLYNN, Monday, September 22, 2014

Quick little update.

We got to the hospital at 8 a.m. Took forever, but I got the port placed in my chest. There was an incision on the side of my neck and one above my chest, and they somehow fed the device through and have it all set up. My neck is crazy sore and it hurts to swallow, which is lame. My chest and neck are all bruised too. Blah blah whatever, it's done.

Just got put in bed. They're pumping anti-nausea stuff into me right now, and then hydration fluids for two to three hours, and then a bunch of other crap. And then other crap on top of that crap. I've absolutely lost track of all that is going to be IV'd today. BUT…

I got placed into the experimental drug group! Very good news for a couple reasons. One is that my doctor is super excited about the chemo drugs I'll be using, as she believes it will be the norm very soon, and that hopefully I'll be a patient that helps further this cause. Also, I won't have to come in on Tuesdays on my two rest weeks for chemo like I would have on the old plan. The Tuesday drug is the one that gives you the most nausea too, so I'm avoiding that all together. So now it's three chemo drugs Monday and Tuesday, two chemo drugs Wednesday through Friday… and then I go in Saturday for a shot and some hydration fluids. Followed by two full weeks of just resting. Excellent.

So anyway, we won't get out of the hospital tonight until 10 p.m. at the earliest, as we were just notified that I got put in this experimental group which calls for more chemo today. But I'm just happy to get started.

I'm just one big walking disaster of pain. I have my left arm taped from having an IV in it during my port surgery. I have my chest all taped up from the port surgery. I have my right arm bandaged from my blood draw. I still have my stitches on my hip, and am walking with a limp from my testicular cancer surgery. I look like a mummy, all wrapped up. Oh, and, I just bit my tongue eating a granola bar… #BestDayEvah

Thank you everyone for all the texts and messages this morning wishing me the best of luck, and sorry I haven't had the time to reply to all of you individually. This is the first minute mom and I have had to breathe here… and I'm about to be fed some Benadryl to knock me out. I really like reading all your comments here… I read every single one.

I'll check in tomorrow after I've had a day of chemo in me. I'm so happy that my cancer is about to get SUPER PISSED about chemo moving in and cleaning house. Haha, what a sucker.

-Ironman

Favorite Comments

Hey! The fast growing cancers are the ones that tend to be most vulnerable to attack. I guess they put all their experience points into offense and none on defense, so if you can avoid their one-two-punch, this boss should be totally beatable. -Navi
—Scott Deeney, September 23, 2014

One down. Next.
—Mark Foss, September 23, 2014

Praying and visualizing each drop of chemo knocking the socks off of those cancer cells! Blessings to you and your mom for a peaceful and good night's sleep.
—Nancy Bohline, September 22, 2014

Ironman,
Glad to hear you are trucking along and so pumped your cancer is about to be super pissed, I never liked cancer. Kick it's ass!! Thinking and praying for you buddy.
—Kali Kasprzyk, September 22, 2014

Is this a bad time to challenge you to the ALS ice bucket challenge?
—John Feldman, September 22, 2014

Way to go Ironman!! Do you glow in the dark yet? Keep your sense of humor!!
—Mary Jo Jasper, September 22, 2014

9-23-2014: Day Two of Chemo

by ERIC GLYNN, Tuesday, September 23, 2014

Sittin' in my chemo bed again. I seriously get like four liters of fluids pumped into me a day. According to my Minnesota math, that's like two-two liters of pop. That plus my five energy drinks during chemo = a lot of pee breaks. Pretty awesome, huh? I actually got placed into a suite today, which has a bathroom and sink, a comfy chair for mom to sit in, and privacy, which is nice. Got here at 9 a.m., and should get out of here about 6 p.m. or 7 p.m. Bah.

I feel literally no nausea or loss of appetite yet, which is good. That actually is supposed to start this evening or tomorrow, so I'm still assuming the worst. All that sucks is my chest and neck from yesterday morning's surgery. I was laying in bed last night like, ok, my surgery from a week ago was on my left hip and side, today's surgery was the right side of my neck and chest… so I basically had to sleep like Dracula. I'm probably about as pale as him at this point too… and I feel a Transylvanian accent coming on… maybe that's just the drugs…?

Hmm, nothing much else to say. Oh! Except below are a couple pictures with my two nurses who will be working with me during my 12 weeks of chemo. Celia is in dark blue. Imelda (I call her "I" cuz I always forget her name) is in pink. They're both awesome and handle my playful, sarcastic jackassness very well. :)

Right now I feel really strong, really determined. Cancer can suck it.

Favorite Comments

Eric, I'm glad you can have such a great "in your face" attitude for the cancer. I'm sure its intimidated.
—Greg Yetzer, September 24, 2014

Your nurses look like the perfect pair to handle your antics. :) Keep up the good fight! :)
—Anne Simon, September 24, 2014

Eric, whatever profession you choose after you KICK cancer OUT... I hope it will include writing. You are an awesome writer. You are helping people in ways you do not even know.
—Pam Traeger, September 23, 2014

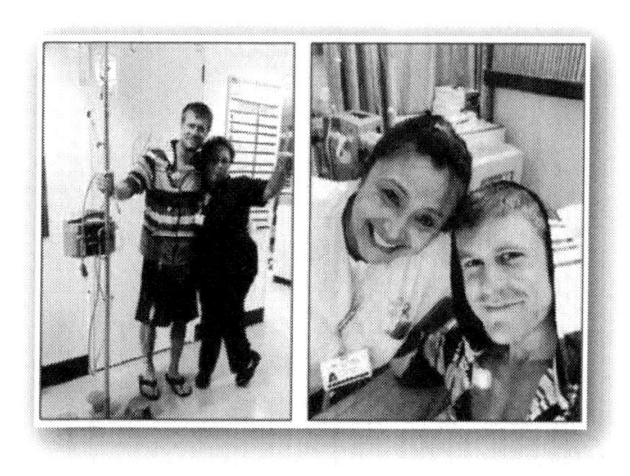

9-24-2014: Side Effects

by ERIC GLYNN, Wednesday, September 24, 2014

It's actually kinda funny, but mostly not... my last post yesterday, I said I haven't felt any nausea and chemo is awesome and blah blah blah... about ten minutes after I posted that I had to call a nurse and get some nausea meds IV'd to me STAT 'cuz I was feeling gross. And the nausea kinda carried over all night too. Probably slept three good hours because I was nauseous the rest of the night and morning.

I also have the driest mouth in the history of mouths. I went and brushed my teeth this morning and when it was time to spit the toothpaste out, it was barely liquid. I was basically blowing sand and dust out of my mouth. So that's pretty awesome.

Hmm, what else? My sense of taste is weird. I had a chocolate ice cream dilly bar thing last night, and it tasted like drinking orange juice right after brushing your teeth. Struggled through it. Chips taste like cardboard. HOWEVER, my energy drinks taste better than ever.

Redbullllllll!

... Speaking of, though... I just had the nutritionist stop in and she gave us a bunch of tips on what to eat and drink while chilling with cancer in your body, and to help with nausea and exercise with cancer and all that, and she poopoo'ed my overconsumption of energy drinks. Kinda funny because we went to Ralph's Grocery last night and I got 10 Amps for 10 bucks and 10 Rockstars for 10 bucks, along with two 4-packs of Redbull. Needless to say, I'll be consuming all this because it's paid for, but I guess I have to slowly taper off energy drinks. That will easily be the hardest thing I've ever had to do in my life, LOL... if you know me, you know I'm not joking.

Currently sitting in bed with about two to three hours left of chemo today. Feeling okay right now. I'll get another shot of anti-nausea stuff before I leave, and then I have a pill I can take every eight hours to get me through until the morning. We'll be home before the sun goes down for the first time this week, so that will be nice. Oh, and, I have a hot video game date with my brother and our friend. It'll be nice to take out some cancery-chemo aggression by shooting aliens for a while.

I'm overall handling chemo better than I thought I would... through two-and-a-half days anyway. Overall, my body is such a wimp but maybe it's going so well because you all are amazing and helping me out a lil' bit? Maybe. ;)

Today's picture is of my two case managers, Elysse and "Purple." Yes, I call her Purple. They both rock.

P.S. I look like a freakin' goof in the picture, I don't know what was happening there...

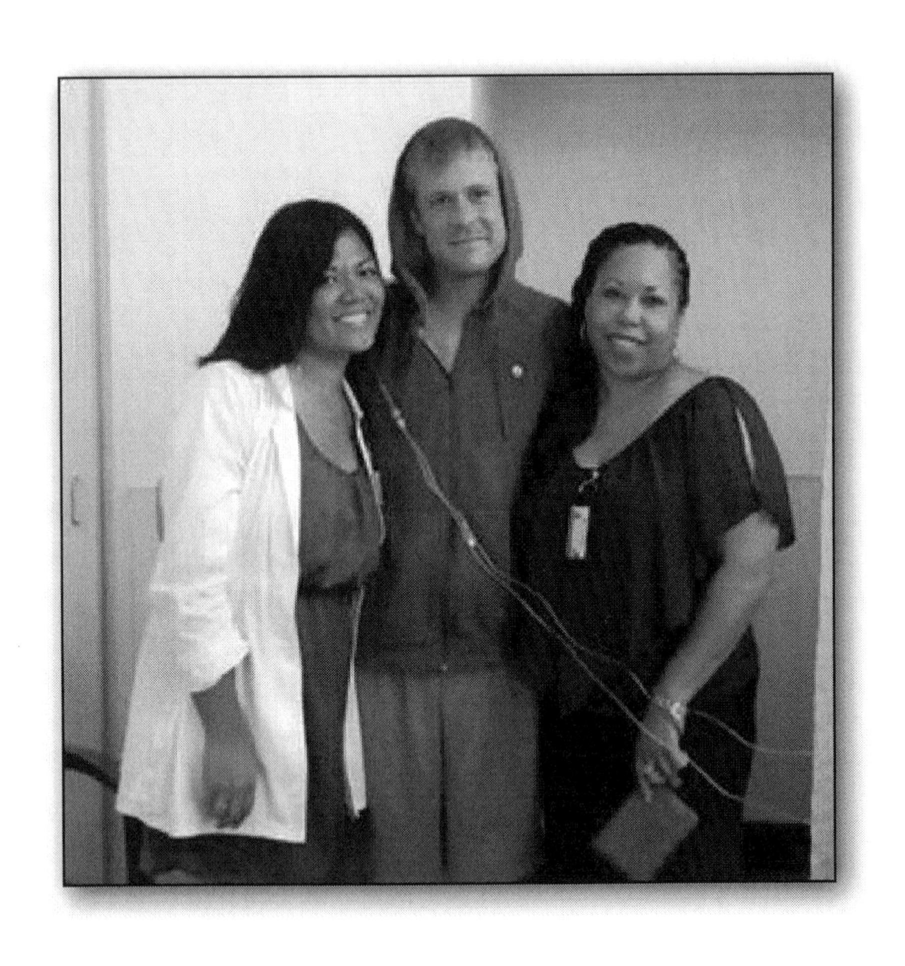

Favorite Comments

Your body is a wimp, only because of the cancer. Your spirit, however, is something else entirely. Build on that. It will help you through. Straight ahead. Everything else is just a detour.
—Mark Foss, September 24, 2014

You're right. You do look like a goof! Oh wait, did I say that - oh no, not gramma! Shoot, the truth is you look like Er!! Sounds like you're doing good. Hang in there. You are definitely not alone and no maybes about it!!
—Anna Glynn aka gramma, September 24, 2014
You are doing great… keep it up! Sounds like you are an awesome patient and I am sure, keeping those nurses laughing... hi to your mom for me.
—Shelly O'Brien, September 24, 2014

You are stronger than you think! I love how you don't have the "why me" attitude, but instead have the "try me" attitude. That will carry you through all this! We are all here for you and are rooting for you all the way! Keep it up! ;)
—Sarah Johnson, September 24, 2014

9-25-2014: Time Flies When You're...

by ERIC GLYNN, Thursday, September 25, 2014

Ok, so I'm not having fun, but time is kinda flying here when I think about things. It's already been three weeks and one day since I was diagnosed with cancer. It's already been two weeks and one day since my first cancer surgery. My mom has been out here for two weeks and two days. It seriously feels like I've known about the cancer for like 72 hours. It's so weird.

Now, it has been a long three-and-a-half days of chemo. That pace has been about right... bah. More side effects. Taste and smell couldn't be weirder. I sleep maybe two to three hours straight at night, but am mostly awake with nausea or shaking. We're getting even stronger nausea meds to take home with us tonight, so that should also help with the sleeping.

It's crazy how fast I get drained. I was ready to rock and do some Target shopping right after my chemo yesterday. I was pumped to get a foot stand and little coffee table of some kind for my video game setup in the apartment bedroom here. Buuuuut, by the time I got out of the car in the Target parking lot and made it inside the store, I was already down to a snail pace and was just like, "Gahhhhh... grab whatever, let's get outta hereeeee." And then I took a nap at home. So yeah, if you come out to visit me, no, I don't want to have a footrace or arm wrestle or swim in the ocean. I sorta want to live through this... ;)

About three hours left of chemo today, and then a full day tomorrow, and then two straight weeks of NOOO CHEMOOOO. But, I guess the worst of the cycle is about to come. So the first five days are when I get my chemo, days 1 through 5 (duh). And I guess days 7 through 10 are when my white blood cells would be the lowest, and I'd be the most susceptible to getting the flu or other garbage. So if I weather through until next Monday, Tuesday or Wednesday, and I'm ok, then I've truly gotten through the worst of my first cycle. And then three more of these bastards. And then hopefully chemo can suck it, surgery can happen, surgery recovery can happen, and then I can be a normal kid again. Yesssssss!

Favorite Comments

I appreciate all your honesty in your posts, Eric. Remember, take only one day at a time, and hug your mother! She is one strong faithful woman who will keep you going. Again, you are in my prayers!

—Cathy Deeney, September 26, 2014

Dude... I know what you can do in your next step of life... write a book! I'll insert some of my depressing poetry from days of old throughout, just to give it a bit of a serious spin. ;) Love you and am praying for you.

—Anne Yetzer, September 25, 2014

You are a splendid writer... I hope you realize that you have that gift.. I am praying for you every day... stay strong mentally and go ahead and ask for help from God and all us out here. Ok?

Mama Foss

—Chris Foss, September 25, 2014

This may be the only time I could beat you in arm wrestling. Actually I bet you'd get tired but you'd still beat my asssssssss.

—John Feldman, September 25, 2014

You have an incredible mindset, Eric. You can get through anything with an attitude and mind like yours. Love you!

—Karen Feldman, September 25, 2014

9-27-2014: Chemo Week One Done

by ERIC GLYNN, Saturday, September 27, 2014

So, good. Five days already in the past. I get my shot today which is supposed to bring on bone pain for a couple days (sounds nice), and typically these next four days are the days that my immunity is the weakest and I can get the flu (sounds nice), but then I should hopefully turn a corner by mid-next-week and at least feel okay for a week or so. I'm definitely due for an okay day. What was your Friday like? Oh, me? ...

10 a.m. to 4 p.m.: Drank chemo
5 p.m.: Ate eggs and toast
6 to 6:59 p.m.: Slept, then woke up running into the bathroom because I thought it was an emergency (false alarm)
7:05 p.m. to 8:04 p.m.: Slept, then woke up running into the bathroom because I thought it was an emergency (half true, half false alarm)
8:15 p.m to 9:08 p.m.: Slept, then woke up running into the bathroom because I... well you get it. Repeat that about seven more times and here we are at 3:40 a.m. my time.

What else, what else. Oh, whenever I eat or drink anything my heart goes insane. It starts revving like crazy. I'm always starving and certain foods taste so good, but I also feel sick as I eat them. The starving part always overcomes though so I get it down. I'm jinxing myself right now by saying this, but I haven't thrown up yet. Gah. I should not have typed that.

Oh, and, the one side effect you're all waiting for............... I still have my hair. Though every once in a while I grab a little handful and see what happens. Nothing has been out of the ordinary yet. It's inevitable that these gorgeous dishwater blonde locks will come out, but it may be another week or so. Trust me, you'll get the unfortunate selfie of that right here when it happens ;)

Favorite Comments

Not to make light of your week, or even your day, but I have to say you write with such humor and irony and wit. Are you by any chance a writer? If not, you should be. Praying the bone pain and flu-like feelings become nothing but a nasty rumor that has no basis in truth! Amen. Take THAT stupid cancer!

Anything we can do to help in the meantime? I know that sounds stupid, but we don't know what you need, but we are nearby, so we can be there in a flash!
—Wendy Housholder, September 27, 2014

9-28-14: Bittersweet... Well, Mostly Bitter

by ERIC'S MOM, Sunday, September 28, 2014

When I first told Eric about CaringBridge, I knew it would be perfect for him because he loves to post and post and post to Facebook, Instagram, and who knows what else. I also thought it would be fun for me to make some entries in his journal from more of a medical and "mom" perspective. I wanted "in" to his journal settings right away, and was excited to get started, but Eric said, "No........... not yet."

Well, "yet" just arrived, and I am not excited at all to write this. And I am feeling a bit nauseous about it. And my heart aches. And tears are falling. And this is not fun. Eric wanted me to send an update to tell all of you that he is getting your messages, texts and calls, and though he enjoys reading them and appreciates the support, he just is not up to responding right now. Here's how bad it is: he's not even turned the TV on for any football!!!! Not even to have it in the background for a wakeful moment. This kid is a fantasy football freak and commissioner of his league...

Eric has spent most of the last 24 hours sleeping. He has been good about drinking water, and has eaten a few things. It's funny what he asks for when he wants to eat. I figured it would be crackers and soup and toast. But no, it's, "Mom, could you make me a cheeseburger, please?" I will go to the ends of the earth to get him whatever he will eat at this point. One of his friends gave him an LA Bite gift card, where they have a relationship with many different restaurants and drivers all over LA who deliver food to your door. What a great idea! Hello, do we have that in Minnesota... where it's cold and snowy? I will have him peruse that site for cravings as he gets better.

He still gets very easily light-headed and heart-racing and nauseous with very little movement, but was able to shower today. Highest temp was 99.2, so that is good. Even though Eric was too blah to watch football today, I'm hoping he is up for "Dancing With The Stars" tomorrow!

Hugs all around! Erix... LOL on this darn laptop my finger always hits the "X" and not the "C" and then it says "Erix" and then I think of Eric and his close friends. They all call him Erix in a goofy voice... some kind of loving nickname I believe.

Eric, if you're reading this, text me your dinner order.

Love, Mom

Favorite Comments

Oh Eric, I'm so glad that your mom is able to be with you and help, it's probably comforting for you that she's there, but it's also comforting for us miles away that she's there!!!!
—Cindy Weber, September 29, 2014

Michelle and Eric,
My heart breaks for you and Eric. Your comment, the tears are falling, as a mother, I feel your pain. Thank God you are able to be with him. Nothing like having your mom by your side. Eric, you are in my thoughts and prayers everyday. I have many prayer warriors here in Illinois praying for you. What you are going through right now is awful. Fight, fight for your health, fight for your life, fight for your dreams.

California dreaming... going to the beach, finding a beautiful girl inside and out to go on a date with, that Ferrari ride down the coast, the warm sunny days while the rest of us will be freezing in Minnesota or Illinois winters. Visualize the life you want and make it come to fruition!
—Lynn Booher, September 29, 2014

What would we do without our moms? Our prayers are with you all, always.
—Cindy Goldenstein, September 29, 2014

Michelle - it's so good that you are there with him... please know my heart aches with yours and all you are going through, too. Hang in there girl, you are a hard working angel like our funny icon at work... please know Eric and you are in our prayers... it should get better for him soon, right? Oh, and the Vikings had a great game… and won!
—Roxy McGraw, September 29, 2014

9-30-2014: I'm Baaaaackkkckckkkkkckckkk

by ERIC GLYNN, Tuesday, September 30, 2014

I can't even describe what Saturday, Sunday and most of Monday were like. Here I'll try, and then we can move on…

I've said it to a couple people already, but I wouldn't wish any of that on my worst enemy. When they say you'll get nauseous and tired… it just doesn't even… those just aren't even the right words. You are nauseous not because you have the flu or because you just went on a rollercoaster and you're dizzy from all the turns. You're nauseous because you can FEEL that there are chemicals inside you and you know your body wants them out. You can feel them, smell them on your skin, in your hair, in your urine even. I didn't move from my bed for three days except to go to the bathroom or to sit up to eat something. Literally. For the first time in my 10 years of playing fantasy football, I didn't watch a game on Sunday. I could have had the bedroom TV on mute and taken glimpses between naps, but I couldn't even look at the screen without thinking I would throw up. Same went for my laptop and cell phone.

And tiredness. I was shaking and getting exhausted eating soup. (I was shaking due to tiredness, mom, promise…

not because the soup was disgusting — my mom makes legit chicken noodle soup.) I had to sit down in a chair right after a shower because I was blacking out. I didn't do stairs for a couple days because I didn't want to fall and put my head through our wonderful host's drywall.

Oh, and incredible bone pain from the shot I got Saturday. Hands, feet, back, shoulders. I couldn't even eat some foods because of the bone pain in my jaw and neck. Lame.

In conclusion: Saturday, Sunday and Monday... yuck. Todayyyyyyyy...

I'm 1000 percent better. Got up and could make myself a bowl of cereal. I actually went outside in the sun for the first time in days and got to walk a couple blocks just to stretch out. I EVEN got to boot up my Xbox One while mom was grocery shopping and kill some monsters and stuff for a while. Kinda dizzy playing, but I'm training up so I can play online again with Bryan and Brandon tomorrow.

Mom is making spaghetti right now, and I'm hungry for it. Yessss. If I am fortunate to have a really bad weekend after my chemo weeks followed by days like today between now and when I start my next cycle of chemo, I will be a happy, happy boy.

One thing I've been asked about a bunch is if I tried smoking pot to help with the nausea over the last couple days. No, but almost. A few days ago I was at my worst, nausea-wise, so I found a number for a medical marijuana facility close by and asked them what I needed to do to get access to some. Turns out I just need to visit with their physician and explain why I need a prescription.

Mom was pissed that I was pursuing this, but after a quick argument she agreed to call Dr. Dorff and get prescribed a marijuana pill as a compromise. If I wasn't so sick and weak

I'd have said, "Eff that noise," and continued my path to get something smoke-able. But I agreed and we picked some up that day. It's Marinol and I dunno... we're mixing it in with all the other nausea and pain meds, so I don't even know if it's making a difference or not. So that's that.

Anyway, thank you so much for all your Facebook messages, texts, voicemails, journal messages, gifts, etc. I received and read them all, but was just out cold the last few days. Know that every single one means so much to me. :)

Oh, btw... my fantasy football team won by a good 50 points this weekend. It was a blowout. I'm about to write my first team power rankings for the year and... spoiler-alert... my team is ranked No. 1 of 10. ;)

Favorite Comments

Er... you are my hero!!
—Annette Glynn, October 1, 2014

Oh Eric! So happy to hear that you're doing better. So sorry about all you're going through! Here's a chuckle for you: I just got back from my mom's funeral. After the funeral, which I spoke at, I went to the bathroom and my neckline on my dress was kind of bugging me. To my great embarrassment, I discovered I had it on backwards. Oh brother! Love you.
—Mary Yetzer, September 30, 2014

Yay, glad you are back... missed you. If you happen to get a spaghetti face after you devour your moms spaghetti... please share a pic. ;)
—Amy Glynn, September 30, 2014

10-1-2014: More To Change ACD (After Cancer Dies)

by ERIC GLYNN, Wednesday, October 1, 2014

Crazy bone pain today. Picked up some pain killers. Trying to back off the nausea meds because I don't think I need them as much for now, and just focusing on taking care of the pain. But didn't have those this morning, so I was awake from 1 a.m. on. Went for a walk during the sunrise and checked out this whole Americana area more. I got stopped by three security guards for trespassing. Instead of flashing my cancer badge I opted for the Americana apartment one instead. I guess the premises are pretty locked down around here. Private parks and stuff. I guess I'M. SO. FANCY... you already know...

... Who dat, who dat, E. R. I. C...

... I'm an idiot. Anyway...

Got a call from my employer today. It sounds like they will hold my sales position for me through the 13 weeks of short-term disability. After that, I will need to return to work or I will be terminated, placed on COBRA insurance should I want insurance, but would be welcome to apply for a new position when the long-term disability ends, probably in April/May/June. Pretty lame, but inevitable I guess? So I can see what they have available when I finish up all this, but this will also be a true chance for me to look all over the place and see what's out there. I'll officially be unemployed ACD.

Anyone looking for a 29-year-old cancer survivor in April, May or June 2015? Is that too specific of a candidate? I can sell stuff pretty well. And can write good too. And by then I should have hair back. I'm considering all options at this point. ;)

Favorite Comments

Dude, I'm thinking it's time to start our business. Amiright? It's a perfect time frame. I'm aiming to still not have hair then, so you can be the face of the company, and I can be the cleaning staff/supply manager. Sorry about the 13 weeks. It's clear they don't want all the money you would make them. Their loss.
—Anthony Giorgi, October 1, 2014

Yay! I'm so glad Alan will be there tomorrow to help! Eric and Michelle, you both are so good at writing your posts. Remember, one day at a time, and we're all holding you in our hearts and prayers.
—Cathy Deeney, October 1, 2014

After this experience... don't you want to be a nurse?!
—Anne Yetzer, October 1, 2014

10-3-2014: Dodgers!

by ERIC GLYNN, Saturday, October 4, 2014

Awesome, awesome day. I feel great. Like seriously if each cycle of chemo is getting it pumped into me for five days, and then three or four days of feeling like total garbage right after, and then a week-and-a-half of me getting back to anything close to this good and I will absolutely dominate all this. I haven't taken nausea meds in two days, am now off my painkillers and feel totally normal. I can't believe that only a few days ago I was struggling so badly.

I felt so good, in fact, that I went to the Dodgers playoff game this afternoon. :) I went with a USC hospital employee and new friend, Elysse. She allllllmost likes the Dodgers as much as me… haha, okay, she's a Dodgers freak. She embarrassed the crap out of me all game with her yelling. Actually we were both really weird and chanting stuff all game. We lost 10-9, so it was a heartbreaker and our favorite player didn't pitch so well, but it was great. We got to see a lot of scoring, a lot of strikeouts, the teams almost brawled after a hit-by-pitch and Tommy Lasorda threw out the first-pitch from about three feet away from home plate like a badass.

My stepdad Alan also flew in today. Met mom and Alan for a late dinner after the game. So happy he's here as it's great to see another familiar face. BUT. I'm ditching out for Huntington Beach tomorrow to give them some time to… ah… "catch up" ……….

It'll be great to be back in Huntington Beach for the weekend, get some good alone time, see some friends down there and rest. I also have been told that I have a card or two waiting for me in my Huntington Beach mailbox, so I'm excited to get to those as well! Thank you so much for all the love and support, y'all. It helped the 'ole spirits during the bad days and is fun to revel in during the good ones. :)

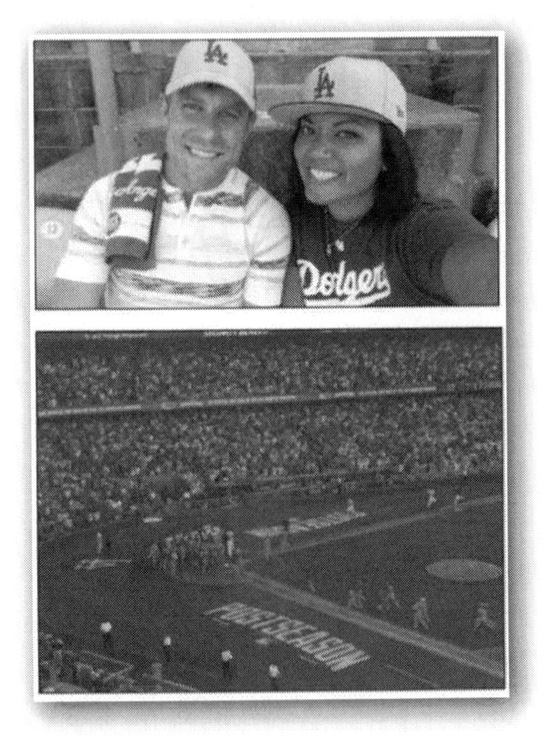

Favorite Comments

Wow!! You continue to be a great example of what positive attitude and a little Ironman will can do!! Enjoy!!
—Cindy Goldenstein, October 4, 2014

So great that you are feeling so well, so quickly!! That kick butt attitude is helping you through! Keeping you in our prayers.
—Leah Hobbs, October 4, 2014

10-4-2014: Bzzzzzzzz

by ERIC GLYNN, Saturday, October 4, 2014

So, after my shower, I came downstairs for breakfast. Mom and Alan were on the couch. I said, "Hey guys, check this out," grabbed a good pinch of my hair and pulled it out with no effort. Haha. It was time for a haircut. Enjoy!

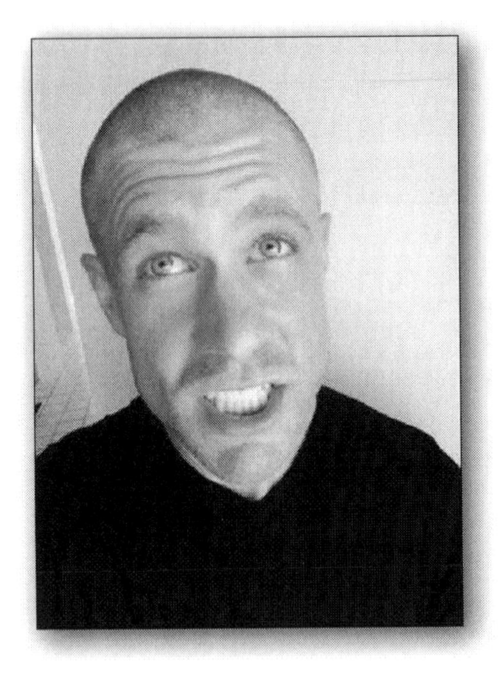

Favorite Comments

I know you have already been battling at the front lines, but you look like a warrior now. Keep up the good fight. We are praying for you continually. Love.
—Greg Yetzer, October 6, 2014

Makes your eyes stand out more... they are gorgeous! Guys do buzz cuts well. Bet mom isn't getting a sympathy buzz.
—Roxy McGraw, October 4, 2014

Instagram 10-5-2015 @eric_t_glynn

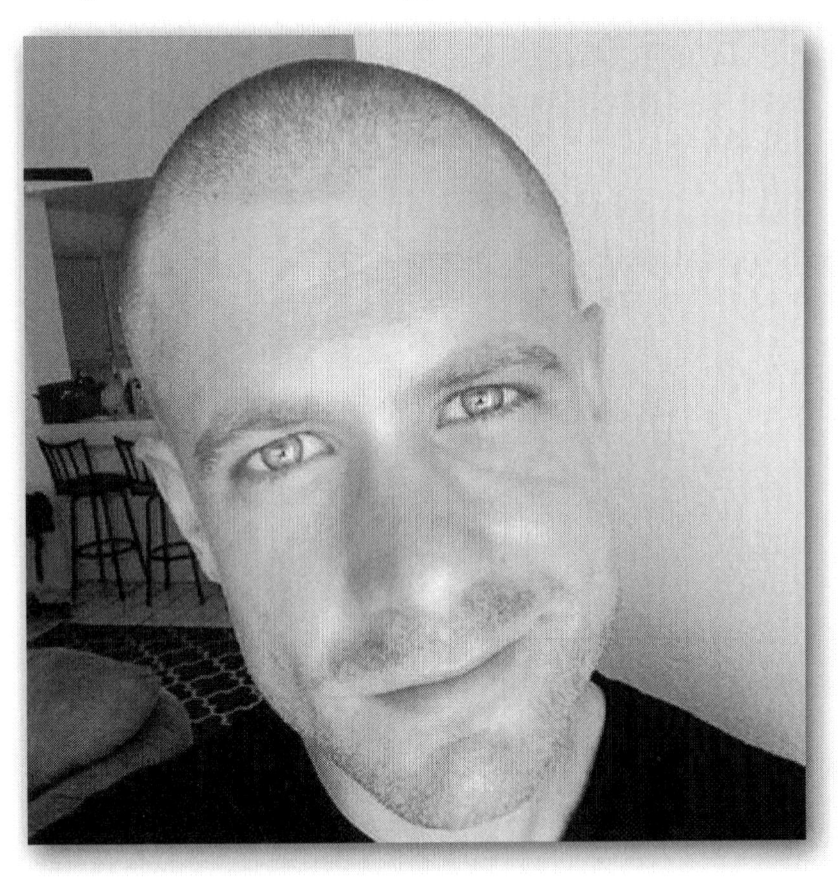

Almost finished with week 2 of 12 of chemo. I'm kicking cancers ass, you guys. There have been some really bad, sick days in there, but right now I feel great. Remember this. Show this to people you know who have cancer or who get it. You're tougher than you know. My caring bridge blog is in my profile. I post in there every other day or so. Take a look, leave comments...you can sign up to get updates when I post a new blog. All the insta love has been INCREDIBLE. You all are amazing people. #douchyselfieoftheday #youretougherthanyouknow #instalove #cancer #chemo #bald #fighter #strongerthancancer #support #loveyouguys

Favorite Comments

@jus***

On my 2nd round of chemo. No fun. I hope you're tolerating the side effects better than me!!!!! #teameric #support #staystrong

@lau***

You look great! I would have never guessed you were fighting cancer! (In fact... I like the bald look on you – very handsome). Keep that smile on your face and that light in your eyes! You will be victorious! :)

@she***

You are my freaking hero <3 <3 <3 I pray you get through this quickly!

@vic***

My grandma and my grandpa are suffering from cancer too. I know how hard it is. I hope and pray you're going to kick cancer's ass, cuz I know my grandparents won't. You are young, you are awesome. Keep on fighting! :)

@11y***

What an inspiration you are. I've lost 3 people in the past 2 years to cancer. Cancer seems to be everywhere we turn.

@rox***

Keep up the positive attitude. Trust me, it will help you through. #survivor

@gib***

Total inspiration... you got true grit and a real spirit.

@tal***

Congratulations man! Your story is simply fantastic. Keep fighting. I'm rooting for you!!

@gaz*****

Hey dad (@algarman1) this guy is also dealing with cancer and keeping a blog of his journey. You guys could inspire each other!

@gre*****

You are doing great! Happy to hear you are doing better!!! Xoxo from Italy!

Random Instagram Stuff

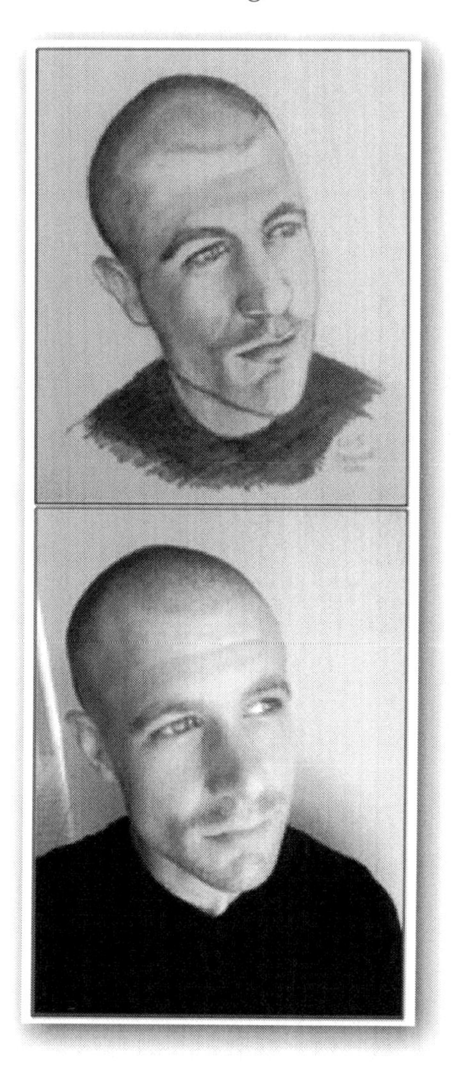

Gretchen Ford (@harleyquinjester99) took the picture on the top off my CaringBridge blog and sketched this for me.

10-6-2014: Feeling Good ^_^

by ERIC GLYNN, Monday, October 6, 2014

What a great weekend. Dodgers game and Alan flying in. Headed back down to Huntington Beach for some good alone time Saturday. Delicious lunch with Tony and Teresa on Sunday and watched sports all weekend. Caught up with someone I haven't talked to in a long time. It felt like I was 100 percent normal, back home, taking the weekend off before the next work week. I've been off all nausea and pain meds for four days straight now. And I get a whole additional week to rest up before chemo starts again on Monday. I feel like you all think I'm faking it because I'm having such a damned good time. Trust me, I'll get "back on track" come Monday, don't you worry... ;)

I also thought a lot about what I want to do while going through chemo. Stuff to do while lying in bed for eight hours of IV awesomeness a day.

So I have a bunch of pictures of SoCal landscapes, the ocean, beach, sunsets, foliage, and then some Minneapolis shots as well... and they're just all a mess in my photo album. I attached a few of my favorites here. I kinda want to clean that all up, group them, make some collages, or group a couple landscape shots together for some portraits and stuff for my Huntington Beach apartment. I have literally nothing on my walls except a portrait of Dwight Schrute from *The Office* (naturally), so it would liven up the place. Could be fun.

This weekend I also wrote about 20 minutes of cancer stand-up comedy that I think may actually be good. I've never done stand-up before, but I think it would be kinda funny to go see a comic who is right in the middle of chemo, bald and stuff, being light-hearted, yet fussy about what he's gone through during chemo so far. Right? My goal is to perform stand-up at least one time during chemo. Haha. Because you only live once.

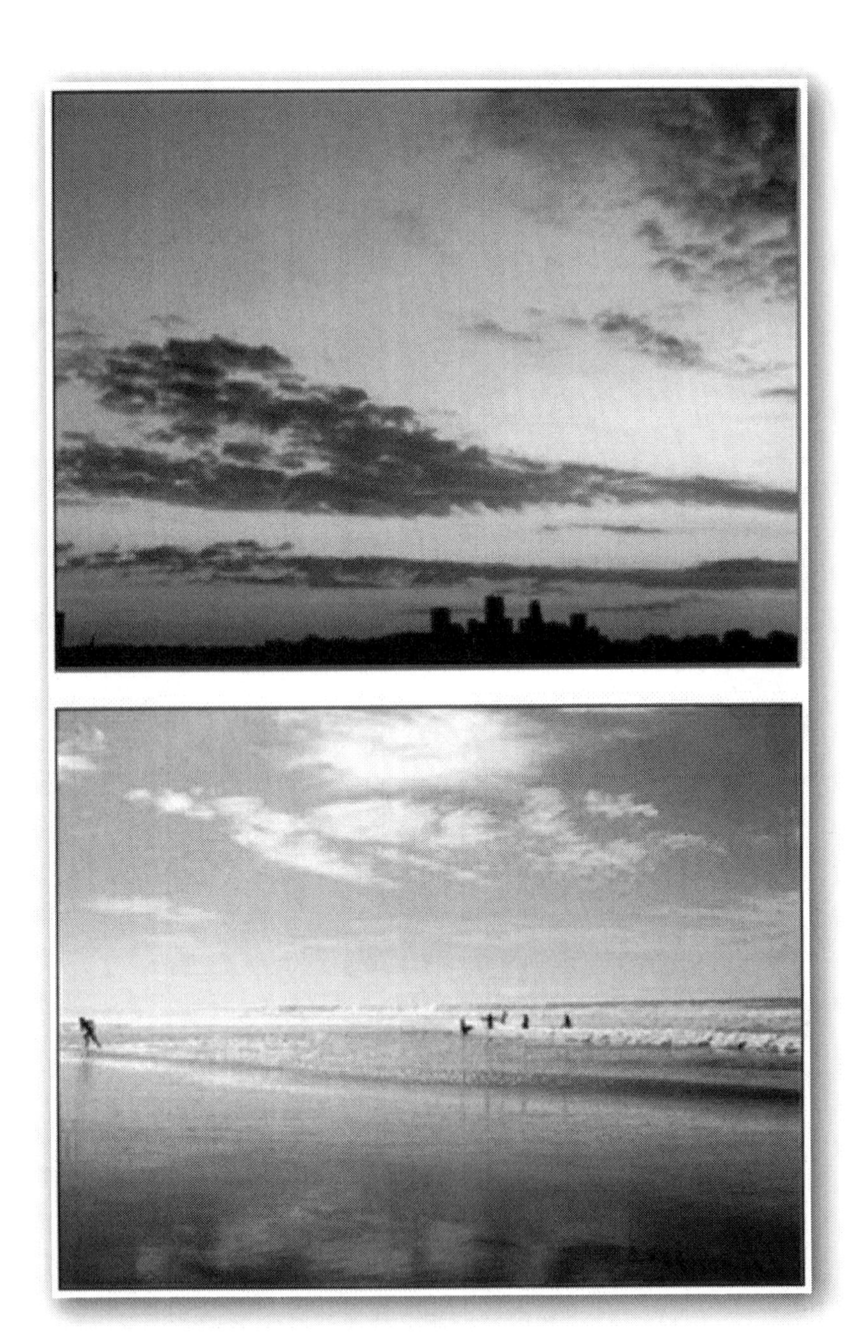

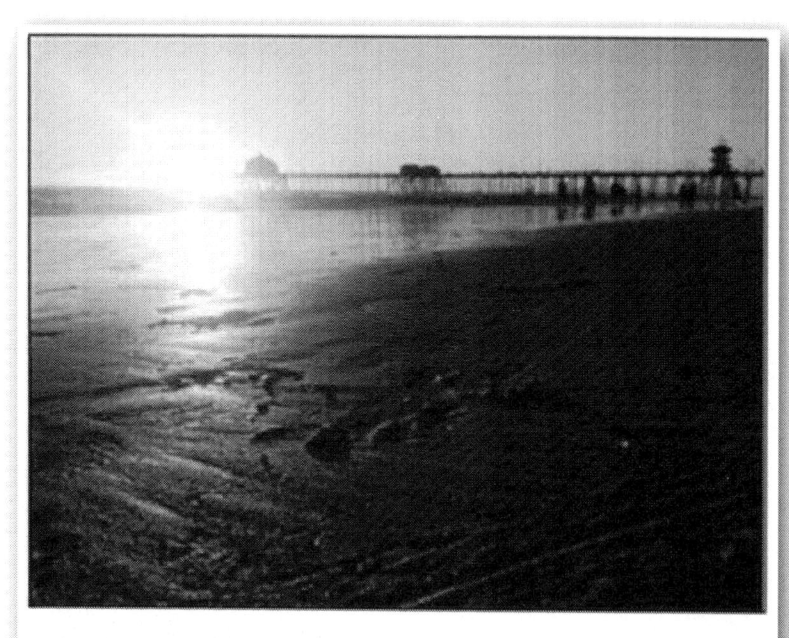

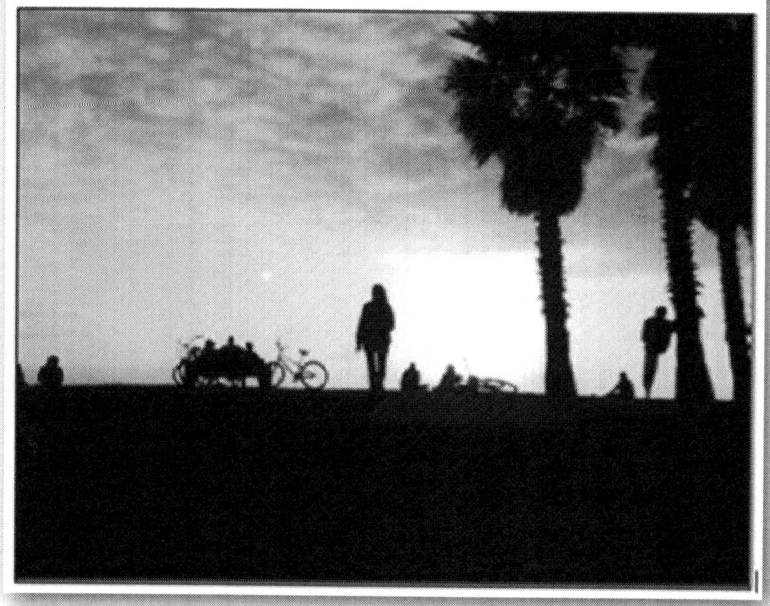

Favorite Comments

I think your stand-up comedy idea is sensational! Go for it Eric! I can't imagine how many people's lives you would brighten! Love you, Mary
—Mary Yetzer, October 8, 2014

Stand-up, I like it... that takes some guts. I get stage fright taking a piss. :)
—Tom Yetzer, October 6, 2014

Love the stand-up comic idea. Be strong and courageous… and bold... and funny… and honest. I'd pay for that performance!
—Kathy Nielsen, October 6, 2014

I think that would be awesome if you did stand-up. Attitude has such healing power and you sharing your story will help heal others.
—Pam Traeger, October 6, 2014

Ummm... I hope I'm not providing most of your material.................
—Eric's mom, October 6, 2014

Eric, I am so glad you are feeling good. Stand-up comedy has been on your bucket list since long before this diagnosis, and I like that you not only want to kick cancer in the balls, you want to make fun of it and also have fun with it. Research has shown that laughter can heal the body, mind and spirit. I will be your audience through this, whether you are on stage or not. Love, Mom
—Eric's mom, October 6, 2014

Love your sense of humor and being able to "live in the moment!"
—Cathy Deeney, October 6, 2014

10-8-2014: First Blood Work Results: Good!

by ERIC GLYNN, Wednesday, October 8, 2014

Yesterday, we went in for blood work to see how the cancer levels and white blood cell counts were doing. And I'm doing well!

You are supposed to see a huge drop in numbers, and we did. Still a ton of work to do as these are supposed to be in the single digits, but…

-The normal AFP number should be 8.3, and I dropped from 1982 to 1014.
-The HCG normal is 0.6 and I dropped from 3133 to 197.2!

*These two numbers need to be at the normal range after cycle four of chemo for me to move forward with the rest period, and then surgery, and a typical white blood count should be between 4,000-10,900, and I have 10,080 so I'm killing it there. Means I'm at a lot lower risk for getting an illness because my WBC count bounced back so hard so quickly. So because my WBC is good, we will be able to move onto round two of chemo on Monday.

It turns out I have an allergy to the "T" in the TIP chemo drugs, which causes a rash on my upper arms, shoulders and back. They gave me a pill to help. So, sweet. Three more cycles of knowing exactly when my body is going to have an allergic reaction to something, and what it will do… with nothing we can do about it besides get through it. Yay, science!

Another random fact we found out: Just because I got this cancer doesn't mean I'm any more susceptible for any other type of cancer. Like I'm not going to have to walk around with a facemask on and an umbrella over my head on a cloudy day like Michael Jackson for fear of the sun. I just can't be a moron. Like everyone else. So it's good to know that I don't just have some garbage genes in general who really like cancer. It should be just a one-off thing. I do NOT plan on needing to post in this blog again for anything else cancer-related after my scheduled finish time of April 2015 for this journey. I prefer it be gone for good. ;)

Favorite Comments

Good news!!! Yay! Congrats! Good job on taking such good care of yourself and listening to your body!
—Karen, October 9, 2014

So you're saying you're going to be the same annoying Eric afterwards? Sigh. I thought for sure they'd give you some special drug to help with that. Guess we can't win them all.
—David Slifka, October 8, 2014

Woooohoooooo!!!! I'm doing my happy dance while using my jazz hands!!! May I do it again PUBLICLY when you are cancer free? Great news, buddy.
—Amy Glynn, October 8, 2014

Instagram 10-9-14 @eric_t_glynn

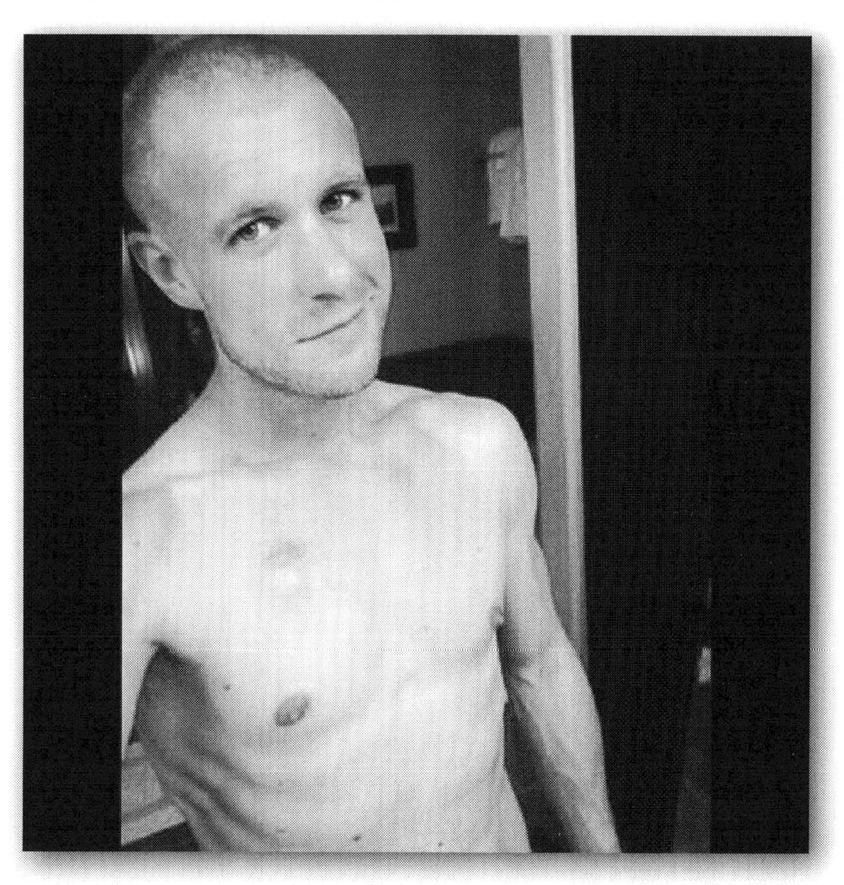

You can see the port they implanted in my chest. That's where they IV the chemo. Due to my age and fitness level my first white blood cell count came back really well so I'll be able to start cycle two of chemo on Monday. (Read more in my blog!) Health and fitness is so important you guys! If you're not where you want to be get started today! #douchyselfieoftheday #cancer #cancersucks #chemo #support #fitness #health #starttoday #loveyouguys #instalove

Favorite Comments

@man***

You seem to have such a positive attitude!! Such an inspiration :) :) Sending positive thoughts your way :) :)

@mar***

Head up man. You're gonna make it through. You have shown how tough you are. Just another obstacle to overcome.

@ms_***

Rooting for you in this fight. I'm going to be saying prayers for you to stay strong until you overcome this, and you will. Just wait and see.

@_it***

Your story is inspiring. I'm so happy you have the courage and strength to share it.

@its***

I stumbled across your profile, looking at lovely cancer-related hashtags. Getting my port put in next week, ugh. Wishing you the best during your fight! :)

@usa***

You're such an inspiration to others who are suffering from cancer. Keep it up and stay strong...

@dis***

Wow, heavy shit. But it looks like you're really fighting back. Stay strong! Lost my dad last year to cancer. You're too young... don't do that.

@ind***

Be healthy, be strong. You're such an awesome dude. Big hug from Indonesia :)

@mod***

I don't know you, but I thought words of encouragement from a stranger could help brighten your day. You're not alone – you got this! And you're awesome.

10-10-2014: Random Hair Update

by ERIC GLYNN, Friday, October 10, 2014

Gah, so even with my head buzzed and facial hair at a 5 o'clock shadow, little slivers of hair have been falling out all the time. I guess I shouldn't be surprised, but I take a shower, get all clean, put on a shirt and it feels like I just got a haircut with all the little annoying hairs all over my neck and shirt.

I was eating ice cream and mom came in and said, "Oh, some chocolate chip ice cream, huh?" ... it was vanilla, but just from chewing the ice cream over the container I got a ton of beard hair into it. Okay, that's gross and didn't happen, but it basically could have.

So I went for the straight clean shave today. I don't know the last time my face was clean-shaven. 2010? Something like that. Literally. Not worth posting a picture of, but I no longer look like I opted to shave my head on purpose due to being in a rock band, but because cancer is up in this bod.

I applied for my California driver's license today. The picture on my license will be my dumb, bald head. I saw the picture. I have a slight smirk, but it overall looks like a gang member mug shot. So after I get pulled over for speeding in my flaming red car, the cop is gonna see this picture and immediately call for backup.

Favorite Comments

Start practicing your stand-up comedy act, as you are seriously good. You might also think about writing a book for patients going through treatment! Your humor would help! Lots of prayers coming your way!
—Joyce Christensen, October 13, 2014

I like how your sense of humor shines through... chocolate chip ice cream might not sound so appetizing for a while?
—Laura Jane, October 11, 2014

I am so glad you have such a good sense of humor about your hair loss, Eric, because honestly sometimes it makes me want to laugh and sometimes it makes me want to cry. It is now outwardly visible that you, indeed, have cancer, and the chemotherapy is doing its job. I am glad I was able to suck an entire vacuum full of your various body hairs, because I think I can knit you a wig to protect you from the California sun, and the Minnesota winter for your trek home to visit… and there will be love in every stitch. :) Love, Mom
—Eric's mom, October 11, 2014

Instagram 10-12-14 @eric_t_glynn

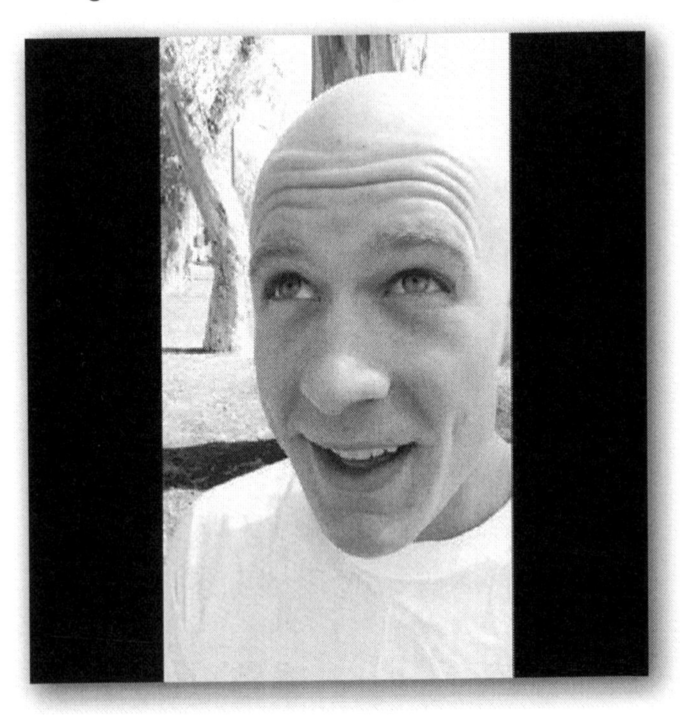

Went for the all out clean shave on the face and the head. It was time. I'm also now healed up enough from my first surgery to where I can do cardio and simple things like push-ups and planks so it's been so refreshing to get back into that. Having an awesome weekend in Huntington Beach with my parents and then back up to USC for round two of chemo on Monday. There are some bad days for sure, but there are some really good days too. Thank you so much for all the comments and the direct messages. I've even seen a couple messages on the Caring Bridge blog in my profile from you IGers. What an awesome support base. Sometimes the coolest comments to read are from total strangers :) #douchyselfieoftheday #cancer #chemo #support #cancersucks #instalove #loveyouguys #superbald #starttoday #fitness #workout #gym #weightlifting #fitfam #weightloss #selfie #cali #california #socal #westcoast #huntingtonbeach #hb #ca #la #losangeles #DMme

Favorite Comments

@bir***

You should be proud of yourself, you're a true inspiration for many, many reasons <3

@nik***

Been reading a little of your posts. You're an amazing guy with such a positive attitude! Thanks for sharing your strength and hope! Hope all goes well.

@kar***

Don't give up. You're an awesome person and also such an inspiration! Stay strong. You can do this! :)

@tes***

I just want to say I wish you the best of luck! My mother was fighting cancer and it was the scariest thing I've ever seen. Sadly she didn't win and only lived for 4 months so I hope that you do kick cancer's ass. Anyone who is fighting cancer I strongly look up to because I believe they are the toughest people out there.

@gen***

You look stronger than ever! It's in the eyes.

@kat***

Unbelievable! You're such an inspirational human being! Keep getting better. Best vibes for your life, you machine!

10-13-2014: Scary Start To Cycle 2

by ERIC GLYNN, Monday, October 13, 2014

Rough start to chemo today. So, the first chemo drug I take on Mondays is the drug that I got the allergic reaction to last week, but it was just a rash. This time, over the course of 30 seconds, I went from feeling totally fine to having my face really flush, feeling like I had a sinus infection, and my throat started closing up and it was getting really hard to breathe. I had to hammer the nurse button to get her in here to stop the chemo and give me some Benadryl. It all immediately got me pretty nauseous, but the Benadryl knocked me out for an hour, and when I woke up I felt okay again. It was pretty scary though. It just happened to have occurred in the three-minute time frame that nobody was in the room so I was like… dammit, guess this is the part where I bite it for good…

But, doing ok now. It's going to be a 7:30 a.m. to 8 p.m. day, and then straight to bed I'm sure.

Yesterday we went out to a nice steak place for Alan's 64th birthday. Happy Birthday, Alan!!!

Also a quick shoutout to grandma and grandpa Glynn on their 60th wedding anniversary!! Love you two!

And to cousin Annie Yetzer's engagement!!!

Oh! Something awesome. Wonderful Ms. Elysse here at USC booked me a stand-up gig. :D :D She has a connection with a San Diego comedian who does a monthly show in downtown San Diego. He said he'd be willing to give me eight minutes of his show in December if I practice at some open mic sessions to figure things out a bit. Absolutely amazing, thank you, Elysse!!

I seriously have 45 minutes of material at this point, so I'll test out the stuff at the open mics and see what sticks and what sucks. And if it all sucks, I'll just go on stage in December and sing Justin Timberlake and Taylor Swift songs in my glorious falsetto.

You can't boo the singing cancer kid… right?

Favorite Comments

Your ears are a lot pointier than I recall. Have you looked into wigs? I could see you with a wig.
—Mike Glynn, October 14, 2014

I'll go brush up on my heckling at a few open mic nights to be ready for that show.
—Justin McMartin, October 13, 2014

10-15-2014: Almost Died Again Blah BlahBlah

by ERIC GLYNN, Wednesday, October 15, 2014

So, I had the same reaction with the chemo drug again yesterday. We fed it to me super slow, but after only 27 milliliters my throat started to close up again and I was feeling flush, so they stopped it immediately and shot me full of Benadryl and steroids to reverse the effects. We eventually tried again, and just like Monday, I was able to handle the rest of the chemo bag. So just another typical day in chemo... near death experience, in the hospital from 7:30 a.m. to 9 p.m. EFF.

Fortunately, the rest of the week consists of only two of the three chemo drugs, excluding the awful one that I disagree with. The symptoms are coming on quicker this cycle. Nausea is starting earlier. Shaking has come earlier. But at this point we have every drug that the pharmacy offers on the dresser at home so I just kinda close my eyes, do eenie meenie miney moe, and randomly pop a few and it tends to work out.

Not much else. Said goodbye to Alan yesterday morning. He'll be back at some point as he left a travel bag here. It was really good to have him out and I hope he saw that mom and I have a good system working here… a surprisingly strategic duo.

Oh! Halloween costume ideas:

-Walter White
-Mr. Clean
-Professor X
-Yoda
-Voldemort
-Charlie Brown
-Uncle Fester… I have to be missing some… help me out…

Favorite Comments

How about a Blue Man Group guy.... hang in there Eric and Michelle! We're praying for strength and peace!
—Julianne Backer, October 16, 2014

Dr. Phil.
—Mike Glynn, October 15, 2014

My vote is Mr. Clean! I know this chemo stuff sucks, but keep your awesome attitude! Laughter is the best medicine!
—Lisa Yetzer, October 15, 2014

Thinking of you. You are amazing, insightful, inspiring... and funny, very funny. Dr. Evil. You could get a Mini-Me doll. Come on - that's a good one, no?
—Lillian, October 15, 2014

Jean Luc Picard.
We could make you a pretty legit conehead. I vote Walter White, though.
—Anthony Giorgi, October 15, 2014

10-16-2014: STL 3 And SF 2 In The Middle Of The 8th

by ERIC'S MOM, Thursday, October 16, 2014

Hi Everyone!

Just want to send a quick update on Eric's behalf. Monday and Tuesday were quite long and scary days, but the last two have gone without incident. Eric got to have his first chemo nurse, Celia, both yesterday and today, and we both just really like her, and Eric especially likes that she gets us out of there by or before 4:30 p.m. :) Eric will admit that the fatigue and nausea hit a day sooner than last cycle, so he's hoping it all ends a days sooner...

We are officially in California, as today we had an earthquake drill. Yes, really. Basically my job if an earthquake hits while Eric is in chemo would be to throw myself on top of him and protect him from falling debris. Eric's job: Sleep through it.

So... I forgot my phone today and noticed it as soon as we got to USC. At first I panicked... I've gotten SO attached to my technology, (believe it or not, Jill.) :) But then I figured it was God telling me he wanted my attention today. Now, how to explain this to Eric so that he believes it was all part of today's plan versus another reason to fire me, or a reason to reduce my CIP bonus (that was for my co-workers.) He said I could make up for this slip up if I watch the Giants beat the Cardinals while he goes to sleep… and that's why the title is the score of the game as I sat to type this. Oh, and now it is tied at 3! Man, should I wake Eric up? If the Giants win the World Series, Eric is set to win a chunk of $ that would be helpful in the coming months, so he is excited for a San Francisco win.

Thank you for your continued prayers and support, and really great Halloween costume ideas. Got one for me since I am the side kick?

Hugs all around!

Eric, drink more fluids!

Love, Mom

Favorite Comments

There is always an extra prayer for the "wing man", errr.... maybe "wing mom?" Keep it up.
—Mark Foss, October 18, 2014

I wasn't thinking duos before. Lois and Stewie from family guy, or maybe Princess Leia and Yoda. Mr. Clean and a cleaning lady. Jean-Luc Picard and Beverly Crusher. Professor X and Jean Gray. Gandhi and Mother Theresa!
—Justin McMartin, October 17, 2014

Michelle, I love your sense of humor! Eric is one lucky young man to have you there with him. :-) My prayers to you and Eric.
—Cathy Deeney, October 17, 2014

I can see where Eric gets his solid personality and humor! Nice update mom!
—Sarah Kneller, October 16, 2014

10-20-2014: "Lame"

by ERIC'S MOM, Monday, October 20, 2014

Eric wanted me to send an update to you, mostly to let you know he is alive, but not well, and he so very much appreciates everyone checking in, and he feels bad that he feels too sick to respond to all the support and encouragement. He thanks you for the words, and also for cards and packages, and if you've not gotten a personal word of thanks, it's coming. And if you've sent a package and not heard from Eric, please let him know as there have been a few sent that never made it, and I know Eric would like to at least thank you for the attempt. :) I smile wondering what we will hear from Justin and Slifka that was sent but never acknowledged...

Since I last wrote, Eric has had some tough days. On his last day of chemo he was uncharacteristically punchy and crabby-ish, and at one point his nurse, Celia, and I had taken enough abuse, so I downloaded Simon and Garfunkel's, "Cecilia" to my phone and cranked it, and Celia gave it her best Miley Cyrus dance and the two of us laughed and danced. We both got an "eff you" from Eric... I'm sure with the greatest affection, and I am sure in that moment Eric regretted that I was becoming so techno savvy. :)

So today, I think Eric is on the mend, and here's how: Three days ago I asked Eric how he was doing, and he asked for a gun. Two days ago I asked Eric how he was doing, and he asked for a gun. Yesterday I asked Eric how he was doing, and he asked for a knife (I'm thinking, "This is great improvement... he just wants to injure himself at this point and not necessarily end it.") :)

Today I asked Eric how he was doing, and he did not ask for a weapon and simply replied, "Lame." Woot!

*For the nurses, doctors, LSW, marriage and family counselors and concerned friends and family reading this: Please understand that both Eric and I have a bit of a twisted sense of humor, and he is NOT clinically depressed or suicidal at this time. Thank you for your concern.

Anywho, I know he feels pretty bad because he did not watch a minute of football over the weekend again! Who filled in as commissioner? Can we get a fantasy football update?

And I know he feels bad because Boyz II Men is playing a free concert in our fountain courtyard tonight, and Eric has no interest in joining me.

And I know he feels bad because he does not want to watch "Dancing With The Stars" tonight.

But honestly, "Lame" is a good thing, so thank you for your prayers and encouragement, and I am sure you will hear from Eric very soon!

Hugs all around!

Love, mom

P.S. Eric!!......Boyz II Men!!!!!! Are you SURE you don't want to join me? We could toss the C-card and get backstage passes!!!! Text me.

Favorite Comments

I would've guessed Boyz II Men was at the point of paying people to come listen. Learn something new every day I 'spose.
—John Feldman, October 21, 2014

The package Eric wants from me I can't put in the mail. Well, I could, but it'd have to be a 6' tall box.
—David Slifka, October 21, 2014

I want you to be my mom, Michelle!!! Love and prayers and prayers and prayers. Eric - you have a mom that will make you mad enough to have the last word – how blessed you are :) Stay strong mama bear and bear cub!

Boyz II Men? Get the gun, friend. Glad you're not calling for lethal objects today. Keep feeling better. Tomorrow will hopefully be 'aight or better. Lots of love.
—Anthony Giorgi, October 20, 2014

Random Instagram Stuff

I got many direct messages on Instagram from followers with their own personal experiences with cancer. This exchange with @kristisue32 stood out.

@kristisue32
I just got entirely sucked into your blog for an hour or so. When I was in high school I took time off to take care of my mom with her cancer/chemo/surgeries. I found myself reading about Neulasta and the sounds of the pumps of the fluids and they instantly took me back. While not all good memories, it was something I hadn't even allowed in my memory in so long. It was a bittersweet trip of nostalgia.

Your mother's writing and attitude warmed my heart through and through and your attitude and outlook makes me smile and eyes swell with tears at the same time.

I'm sure you get a ton of messages but your story and your blog touched me in a way I hadn't felt in a long long time. You're incredibly brave to put it all out there and be so real with it all. When I read your mom's story about pancakes I remember when all I could get my mom to eat was watermelon for days and all of a sudden she wanted a roast! I've never moved so fast to the store in my life :) I forgot about things like that, so thank you. Thank you so so much. You and your family are amazing for doing this and being so real in such a hard time. Stay strong :)

@eric_t_glynn
Well thank you for reading about me! Yes, little things like the sound of the fluids machine and just sitting there for hours and hours… that's stuff I hope leaves my memory too! I hope your mom made it through it all ok? I can't wait to be a success story when this is all over :)
Thank you for the sweet message :)

@kristisue32
You're welcome. Anything to make you smile after what you just blessed me with. And you'll be a great success story. Keeping track of it all will be a gift later in life and you're helping so many people too. My mom unfortunately did not make it, but the whole experience was life-changing and she made me who I am today, even if it was short. I don't want to damper your evening though… positive vibes :) You're reaching and changing so many more lives… amazing.

10-22-2014: Let The Good Times Roll

by ERIC GLYNN, Wednesday, October 22, 2014

I'm backkkkkckkackackakkkckkk... again. Let me catch you up on ALL I've been up to the last few days:

Friday 5 p.m. à Tuesday night: Laid. In. Bed.

There we go. All caught up on my life. I was on my ASS until yesterday evening. But just like the Tuesday after chemo last cycle, I felt a pretty good resurgence yesterday morning. I had pancakes and eggs for breakfast, Chipotle for lunch and New York style pizza for dinner as a big "suck it" to cancer for putting me through those rough days again.

So again, sorry if my responses were scarce the last few days. Reading all the texts and emails, Facebook stuff and Instagram stuff and catching up now. I wasn't playing video games and avoiding you. But yeah if you feel ignored over the next couple days... it's because I'll be playing video games and avoiding you. ;)

So mom and I are in Huntington Beach for a couple days. We jammed to The Cars with the windows down during the drive. I'm currently at Starbucks listening to my favorite Beatles song *(bet you can't guess it)* and mom is taking some alone time for herself. Our goal is to do NOTHING but binge watch "The Voice" to get caught up and enjoy some CTO (cancer time off.)

And then Friday morning, dad and my stepmom, Mary, fly in and will be with me until Tuesday afternoon's blood work visit. They'll get to see the Huntington Beach area and then get up to USC to meet my oncology team. Looking forward to the visit!

Most of the sports world has gone awry in my absence. My fantasy team lost. The Minnesota Wild lost to both LA teams. BUT. The San Francisco Giants are three wins away from the World Series, and a payday for me! I put $200 on them in April to win the World Series, and if they do I get 19x my money back. You got that right, $38,000,000! Right? Errr… less? Something close to $38,000,000, I think…

P.S. "Don't Let Me Down"… kind of an ode to my chemo…

Favorite Comments

Perhaps you did not know it is John Feldman's Poem Thursday.
This week is delight in the form of a limerick.
There once was a man named Glynn
His strength could fill a grain bin
As it attacked his scrote
He did everything but gloat
And he manned up to f&%$in win
—John Feldman, October 23, 2014

Love these updates Eric. Happy that "YOU'RE BAAAAAACK" in action. Enjoy your CTO and more family time. Chipotle solves every problem... well maybe chocolate too.
—Jennifer Dixon, October 22, 2014

Instagram 10-27-14 @eric_t_glynn

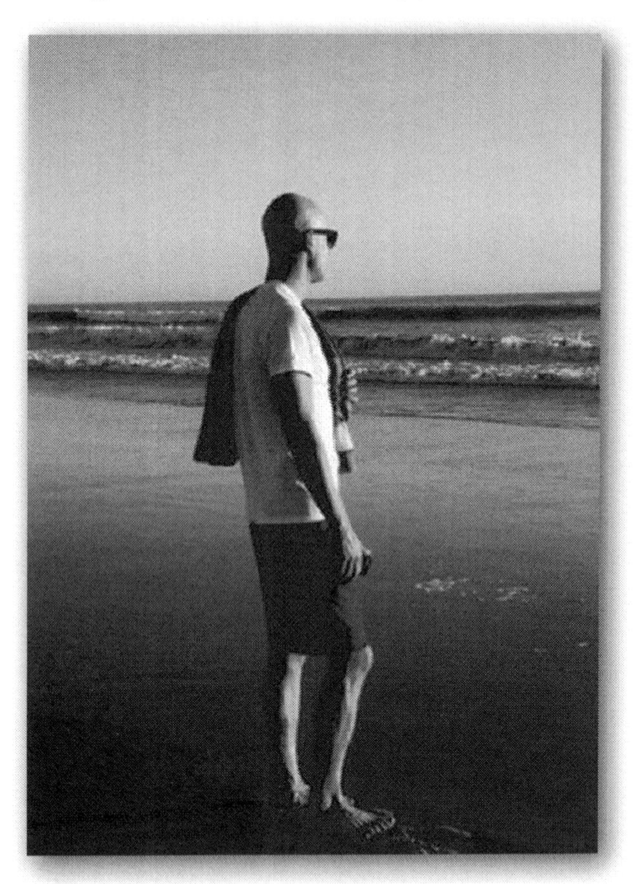

There are some bad days, but there are definitely some good days too :) Just finished week 5 of 12 of chemo. Almost half done! Your support has been amazing. It's great to lay in the hospital bed and get to read your comments and messages of hope. We're almost half done, guys ^_^ #douchyselfieoftheday #youretougherthanyouknow #fighter #cancer #chemo #support #cancersucks #instalove #loveyouguys #superbald #starttoday #fitness #workout #gym #weightlifting #fitfam #weightloss #selfie #cali #california #socal #westcoast #huntingtonbeach #hb #ca #la #losangeles #Dmme

Favorite Comments

@sin***

I have to say, it's amazing how you handle this! Your strength is unbelievable and I can just look up to you! Hope you'll go through the whole process with this courage that you have now! All the best for you!

@ren***

Stay strong and spend time in nature as you are. It will keep your spirit high! Will continue to pray for you.

@adr***

I never comment... but your positivity is incredible. Hugs :)

@nov***

:'(Heart-touching...

@swe***

Hey Eric. I own/operate the Sweetcakes cupcake booth down on Main Street each Tuesday night, and you've been kind enough to like some of our stuff on Instagram. If you're interested in liking how much they taste as well as look, you or your mom can swing by tonight or any Tuesday, and I'll hook you up. I normally wouldn't tempt you if you were on your normal workout/dietary regimen (insanely jawdropping, btw) but if you're eating pancakes and pizza, I figure that's out the window for now.

@lex***

Thinking of you hot stuff! When you're ready, feel free to come down to Melbourne, Australia so I can marry you! #notevenjoking

@kru***

Sometimes I see people who have everything and appreciate nothing. You seem to appreciate everything, even when you have lost so much. Respect.

@kar***

My Godfather just died a month ago from cancer. He was literally my everything, the best. Ever since, I admire people who are fighting it and I love people who stay strong and keep their head up. It's a hard road for you and the people around you, but if you believe you can, then you're half way there. Good luck with all my heart!

@eric_t_glynn

@kar*****Thank you so much for sharing that. I'll fight extra hard to make him proud.

@kar***

You just brought tears to my eyes. That's really a sweet thing to say to someone you don't know. I'll pray for you, and light up a candle right now. Again, good luck.

@lau***

I noticed you commented on my HB sunset photo. Thank you! I also noticed you live in HB and are going through some difficulties right now. This is such a small world. About 8 weeks ago, I drove down to HB after work to watch the sunset. It was beautiful and this VERY nice lady asked me if I thought the sunset was done. She told me she was taking photos for her son who usually posts one everyday, but he was too sick to do it himself. I found out that he had just moved out here for work when he was diagnosed with cancer. I am 99.9% sure that that lovely lady was your mom! I prayed for you that day and have thought about your mom. I'll keep you in prayer! Tell your mom "Hi" from the lady from Anaheim :)

@eric_t_glynn

@lau***** That is absolutely crazy. That sounds like my mom alright ^_^

10-28-2014: Dad And Mary Visit, Latest Blood Work

by ERIC GLYNN, Tuesday, October 28, 2014

Sup. Just had a great long weekend with dad and Mary. We were just three crazy kids renting a three person buggy bike, watching surfers, seals and sunsets. Great to see them. We made dad eat sushi, made Mary eat buffalo wings, and made me eat oysters. All against our will. Oysters can suck it.

Looks like Kansas City is up 7-0 in the 2nd inning here, so this will go to Game 7. **DON'T BLOW THIS, GIANTS. I HAVE CANCER FOR GOD'S SAKE…**

Dad and Mary got to meet the oncology team today, and we got some updated blood work numbers:

—The normal AFP number should be 8.3, and I dropped from 1982 at the start to 1014 after the first cycle to 228 today.
—The HCG normal is 0.6 and I dropped from 3133 at the start to 197.2 after the first cycle to 7 today.

*These two numbers need to be at the normal range after cycle four of chemo for me to move forward with the rest period and then surgery, and a typical white blood count should be 4,000-10,900, and I have over 11,000, so my body rocks and I'll be able to start cycle three of chemo on Monday.

So all good news. Cancer's balls are being kicked.

Just dropped the 'rents off at the airport. Back in Huntington Beach for some alone time until Friday afternoon, and then bringing mom back to paradise for the weekend.

Booya.

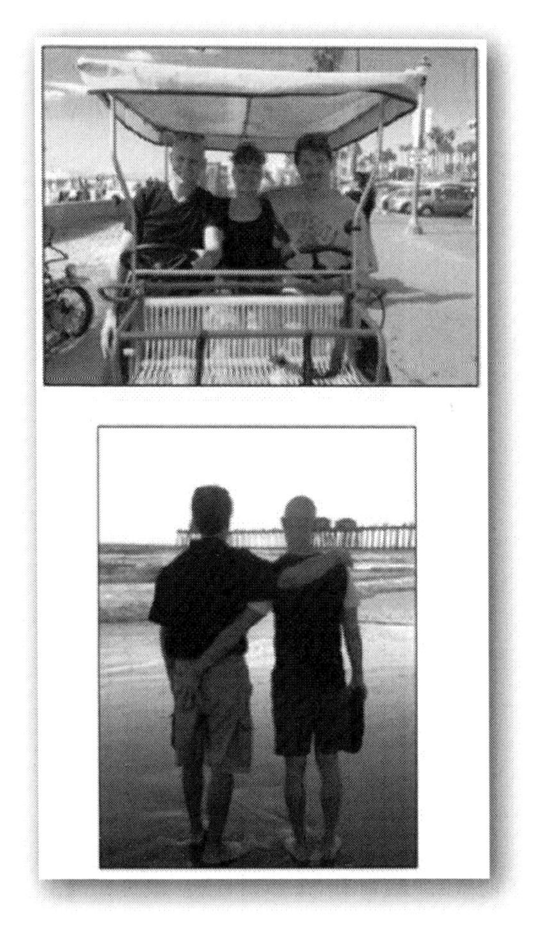

Favorite Comments

Fabulous news bud!!! So great to see the pics of you, dad, and Mary. Sounds like you guys made the most of your time!!! Bet it was hard for father to leave son... ughhhh!! Made me want to be there so much just to hug the stuffin' out of you!! Love you bud.

—Amy Glynn, October 29, 2014

Great news Er... love the sunset pic with pops on the beach. You make a lovely couple.

—Annette Glynn, October 29, 2014

Congrats on your labs Eric!! Don't worry the Giants can make it happen!!

—Lisa Yetzer, October 29, 2014

Alone time and Game 7. That's a good day.

—Mark Foss, October 28, 2014

10-29-2014: No Shave November

by ERIC GLYNN, Wednesday, October 29, 2014

San Francisco Giants won the World Series! Money in the bank! Best year of my life! Well, maybe not… LOL.

Anyway, I have something important to say… for ONCE.

Two of my friends and frequent commenters, David Slifka and Justin McMartin, are participating in "No Shave November" next month, aka "Movember." October is Breast Cancer Awareness Month, and November is kind of a guy-parts cancer awareness month, where men don't shave all month long to show support and collect donations.

They've set up a website to collect donations for cancer research.

There is the link to follow to learn more about "No Shave November," to donate and/or to join their team and opt out of shaving for a month to show support and raise awareness. Whether you opt to look like a caveman for a month or not, please send the link to coworkers, friends, family… these guys have a $1,000 goal, but are already at $285, and November hasn't even started yet, so I think we can blow this number out of the water.

Now, these two guys are pretty sketchy and there's an outside chance that this whole website is fake and that this is actually a Vegas fund for those two jackasses… but don't worry, Vegas is only a four hour drive from here, so if that's the case I'll track them down and cancer punch them in the guy-parts…

Just kidding. This is an awesome cause, a cool way to show support and raise awareness, and I'm excited to see daily updates on how patchy and thin their beards are throughout the month. I don't know if they can post update pictures on the website link above or if they'll post on Facebook, but I'll be sure to attach some update pics on here for you to enjoy.

Justin, David and I will keep an eye on the comments for any questions. I'm excited to see what this cancer team of mine can do!

Favorite Comments

Justin and David, I'd like to join and am seeking the blessing of my work overlords. Either way, you've got my $$. Way to go.
—Anthony Giorgi, October 29, 2014

My mom keeps telling me I'm getting a mustache... I promise not to wax it til December! Maybe other people will start to notice it too and I'll proudly tell them about the cause!
—Anne Yetzer, October 29, 2014

If I can figure out the tech part of making a donation, I plan to join. I will not shave my arms or legs or pluck my pesky upper lip menopausal whiskers for the entire month of Movember!! You will all be grossed out by the update pics I will send. Thanks for setting this up, Slifka and Justin!
—Eric's mom, October 29, 2014

Instagram 10-31-14 @eric_t_glynn

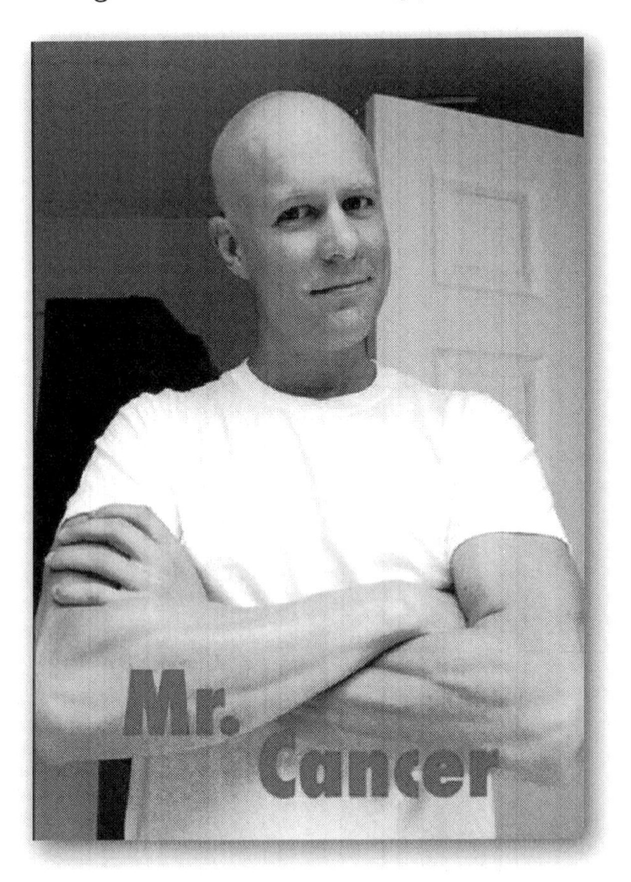

Mr. Clean? Nope, Mr. Cancer! Do a Google Images search for Mr. Clean and let me know if I nailed it or not :) If you can't make light of the dark stuff that comes your way, the darkness will consume you. My Halloween costume was zero dollars and took zero minutes to make. ^_^ For the record I'm awful at cleaning... #douchyselfieoftheday #youretougherthanyouknow #fighter #cancer #chemo #support #cancersucks #instalove #loveyouguys #superbald #starttoday #fitness #workout #gym #weightlifting #fitfam #weightloss #selfie #cali #california #socal #westcoast #huntingtonbeach #hb #ca #la #losangeles

Favorite Comments

@daa***

Good wishes Mr. Cancer.

@tra***

I think you are missing an earring :)

@luc***

I'm from Mexico and I just saw your profile and you really inspire me. I hope you get better and when the cancer ends (I know you're gonna make it) you keep inspiring people. I'm your fan.

@aic***

I'm really impressed by your motivation and your strength for fighting cancer. I wish you all the best from France. Keep smiling :)

@bah***

You are Mr. Amazing.

@l20***

Dude, your ability to find laughter in hell is astonishing. I wish you the best of luck in your fight :)

@onu***

Your sense of humor regarding this is so endearing. It's amazing how we first see the surface, but once we pull back the cover, we discover so much more. Your documentation of your journey is sure to inspire. Major kudos to you! Strong, handsome and resilient :)

@ele*****

Non-Hodgkins Lymphoma survivor here. Keep strong. You've got this!

@kar*****

Sad, but really inspirational. It made my day, thank you :) Best of luck and prayers to you <3

@he*****

I'm reading your story. I love it. I was almost in tears, because of the great amount of strength and courage I was seeing. Then this one made me laugh :) #stupidcancer #dontstopfighting

11-2-2014: Oh Boy, Here We Go Again

by ERIC GLYNN, Sunday, November 2, 2014

Last day in Huntington Beach. Heading up to LA and then up at 6 a.m. to start cycle three tomorrow morning. Bah. I'm sort of over cancer. Is there some store I can return it to? Or can I donate it to Goodwill or something? No? Ok, ok I'll keep it, but only for two more cycles, dammit.

This round will be a little different though because we want to try and NOT have my throat close up and have me die in my chemo bed. We're going to pump me full of steroids and Benadryl today and tomorrow morning so I'll be a walking zombie, but hopefully take the chemo okay. I'll still get the full body rash like I did the first two cycles (gross), but hopefully that will be the only allergic reaction. Oh joy!

Anywayyyyyyyy. I got to have a fun night out being a normal kid with my Huntington Beach family this last week. It was really fun to goof off and talk smack and bar hop a little bit. Can't wait until I can do that again... with hair, someday.

Looking forward to the short-term future though. After this cycle I have Will, John and Tony, my close friends from high school, come out for a weekend, followed by my brothers, Bryan and Mike, the weekend after. Haven't seen any of them in months so it will be great to show them the Huntington Beach area and act like morons for a couple days.

Last thing, and this is a little self-serving. I kind of want to take these journal entries, add some pictures, Instagram posts, texts and turn it into one big cancer memoir, somehow. The title will be "Kicking Cancer in the Balls." Or something like that. I dunno, just throwing the idea around. Maybe it wouldn't be attention-getting enough or just be another cancer book on the shelf and it'll go nowhere, but I'm wondering where to even start. Has anyone ever published a book, pursued publishing a book, know a publisher, editor, agent…just, anything? Worst case, I'll self-publish something and give it to my kid someday… selling one copy to myself, LOL.

Favorite Comments

I'd buy the book, but I might not let my kids read it til they're past age 13. ;)
—Anne Yetzer, November 3, 2014

Your life dude, do what you want. I read one time that a being can do anything, for however long it might take, for as long as he wants to. Please know that we all here are on you journey, supporting your will to do what you really want to do...
Oh, and I'm in for a first edition of that book. Now if I can find my checkbook...
—Mark Foss, November 2, 2014

Selling one copy to yourself, sounds about right for your sales history. Zing! Keep on rocking man.
—David Slifka, November 2, 2014

11-4-2014: No Allergic Reactions!

By ERIC GLYNN, Tuesday, November 4, 2014

So all the steroids and Benadryl we pumped me with the night before and the morning of chemo have worked. No throat closing up for me! Pretty neat, I suppose. The steroids have actually woken me way up, and I'm getting all this work done… calling insurance companies, my employer, the state of California, and stuff like that. It's a good day so far.

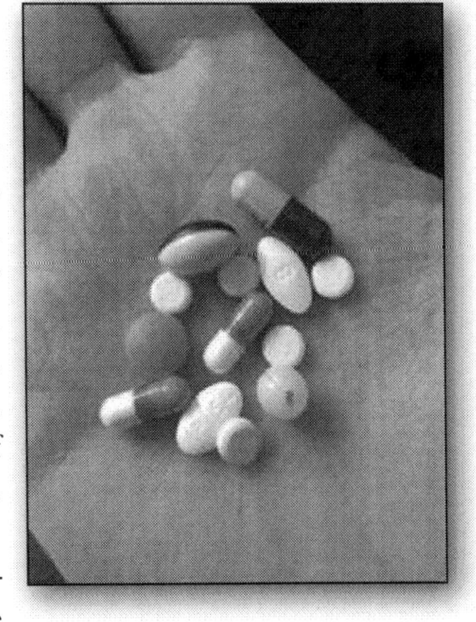

Here's a pic of my "dinner" last night, aka all the pills I've had to take the last couple days. No idea how this didn't cause an overdose.

I did, however, wake up this morning with a runny nose, sneezing, coughing, plugged ears and messed up vision. Like almost blacking out. We did a couple blood pressure tests and my BP while standing was like 84 over 44 which is way off I guess. Just need to take things slow.

Not a lot else to say. Just excited my throat is open and breathing okay. The damned rash has already started again, but there's nothing we can do about that. I don't really have much of a reason to take my shirt off anyway. I'm also about as pale as I've ever been in my life... and my white, bald head and light-colored eyebrows don't help. In conclusion, I'm so hot right now, you guys. Rawr.

Favorite Comments

Your candor and humor is refreshing. You continue to be in our daily thoughts and prayers. So glad the allergic reaction was not like last time. Hang in there... you're doing great!!
—Jill Steinhauser, November 6, 2014

All that just puts more focus on those delicious tractor-beams you call eyes!! Your fan club will always love you regardless- Mwah!!
—Helen Blythe-Hart, November 5, 2014

Cracking me up again!! And YAY!!! That's great news bud!! So happy that colorful concoction worked for you!! Love you sooooo much!!!
—Amy Glynn, November 4, 2014

Hang in there Eric! Your positive outlook is so inspirational! Lots of love, Mary
—Mary Yetzer, November 4, 2014

Glad to hear it's going better this time. Thirteen pills is about the same amount I take daily to stay sane.
—Bill Yetzer, November 4, 2014

11-6-2014: Today Was Brought To Us By The Letter "F"

by ERIC'S MOM, Thursday, November 6, 2014

So, Eric reported to you earlier this week that he was nearing blackouts, and dealing with low blood pressure. Yesterday was worse, and his standing BP at one point was 79/44 with a pulse of 116. Today was a little better, according to the numbers, but not in how Eric was experiencing the day. He felt so bad that he did not think it was safe for a shower and he feels super nauseous today. "F" is for "faint."

We have seen a lot of celebrities during our time here, and this morning it was no different. As we pulled out of the parking garage, there on the sidewalk greeting kids and families at 8:30 a.m., was Santa and Shrek!!!! "F" is for "famous."

Eric noticed that the front of his Mercedes grill was more than a bit discombobulated. Something bad had happened recently, but what? At first he asked if I wanted to make a confession, but Eric has been in the car for all of my near misses. So he made the assumption that the USC valet employees did something to his car, so when we arrived this morning, he was a bit animated (which was good for his blood pressure) and he was taking pictures, filling out forms, demanding video, etc. "F" is for, well, "eff."

When we got to chemo day at the hospital, Eric's nurse, Celia, (who comes in an hour earlier than she needs to just to be sure she gets Eric as a patient, and to make sure he is taken care of immediately upon arrival). Well, anyway, yesterday she had to put him in room J, which I LOVED, because it had a window and it was nice and warm. Eric hated it, because it had a window and it was nice and warm. :) Today Celia made sure Eric was NOT in room J, and instead we were put in room… F. "F" is for "F" in this case.

So for the past two cycles, going in to USC for Neulasta and hydration on Day 6 (Saturday) was horrible for Eric, because generally Friday, Saturday and Sunday are his very worst days. He refused hydration last time because he did not want to spend the two hours there to allow for the infusion, even though he nearly blacked out getting there, which meant he needed the infusion. Well, he was able to talk his oncologist into arranging for the Neulasta shot to be mailed to us, so that I would get to give it to him at home, so he would not have to leave the apartment on Saturday. So now we are dealing with a pharmacy. Family and friends know that I have spent countless hours on the phone and in the waiting rooms of pharmacies all across California trying to keep this child on drugs, so I cringed at the thought of relying on a pharmacy… even though it was a "specialty pharmacy," to get this right. I have been in contact with them every day this week, reminding them day after day what the mailing address is, to be certain it gets here in Glendale, and does not go to Eric's apartment in Huntington Beach. I did not sleep well last night worrying that it wouldn't get here, and we will miss the window of administration for Eric's white blood cell needs and for the research protocol, so I called the "specialty pharmacy" again this morning and they were very sorry, but they had sent it to the wrong address!!!

Since they would not guarantee delivery to the correct address within 24 hours, I made the executive decision to fire the pharmacy. I told Eric we are coming in to USC on Saturday for Neulasta AND hydration, even if I have to call security to put him in the car. We all know what "going postal" is. Well, I think I've coined a new phrase: going pharmacy. "F" is for "fired 'f'armacy!"

So, I got Eric home and in bed tonight, and needed to walk to Target Pharmacy to pick up some meds they PROMISED would be ready for me anytime after 2 p.m. today, and it was now 5 p.m. Yes, I am a glutton for pharmacy punishment. Well, it was not ready AND they only had enough for a day or two, so could I please come back for the rest? :) I took the pills, and decided I better get out of there before I went all pharmacy on them, and so that I wouldn't find myself on the 10 p.m. news with Paul Majors. "F" is for "frustration."

By the time I got home from the pharmacy, I needed a drink! So, I pulled a bottle of wine from my Bevmo case, and when I went to open it, the squiggly cork remover part of the wine bottle opener busted off… before I got the cork out! "F" is for no "fruit serving!"

Three more "F"s and we can all go to bed and try this again tomorrow: Family. Friends. Faith. These three things lift us up, shake us off, fill our hearts and propel us forward. I thank you, and Eric thanks you.

Eric, please wake up and drink more fluids. We will get through this.

Love, Mom

Favorite Comments

Oooh fuuuuuuuuuudge! Only I didn't say "fudge." I said THE word, the big one, the queen-mother of dirty words, the "F-dash-dash-dash" word!
Sometimes, I think it is appropriate.
Mom, let it fly... most here would really understand. Only because of our own frustration...
—Mark Foss, November 7, 2014

I have another word for you two, "FIGHTERS!" Tomorrow is another day, keep focusing on the positives. Sending "faith" your way.
—Jennifer Dixon, November 7, 2014

I am so sorry for the frustration you are going through just to keep Eric on the right path with his meds. As always... both of you are in my prayers.
—Annette Glynn, November 7, 2014

And somehow I forgot FEARLESS–if there would be a definition Michelle your picture would be next to it.
—Cindy Goldenstein, November 7, 2014

F is for Friday!!!! You made it through your 3rd round, only one left!!!! I'm sure you're Frustrated, Frazzled and F-in sick of this!! But know that we all think you're Fantastic, Fearless and so Faithful. :) Forge Forward Fearless Friend and keep the Fluids going (For both of you!!) Loves
—Cindy Weber, November 7, 2014

11-8-2014 : And The Score Is: Eric 3 – Cancer/ Chemo 0

by ERIC'S MOM, Saturday, November 8, 2014

Hi Everyone!

I will let Eric describe the last three days to you in his own words, but I can tell you it has been difficult. Cancer/ chemo got behind Eric a few times and kicked him in the butt, but true to his mission, Eric turned and kicked back... in the balls!

Eric got up and faced the chemo day after day, and today he faced USC again for some hydration to help his strength, nausea and kidney function, and he also got his Neulasta shot which means bone pain ahead. We have armed ourselves with stronger pain meds this round, and are taking it as a prophylactic in hopes of a more comfortable outcome.

Eric, my son. I am so proud of you. I am so sorry when I have to take off my mom hat and put on the coach/drill sergeant hat (I need a whistle!) to be a help to you through chemo week, and the next few days ahead. It might not feel like care and concern in the moment, but while I am refusing to turn the fan back on until you sit at the edge of the bed, please know that my heart is breaking inside for your pain and suffering.

And so, dear friends and family, here is what we need prayer for in the coming days: Eric needs to have the strength and desire to be able to feed and water his good cells while the bad ones are being killed off from chemo. And his bones need to get busy keeping Eric high in WBC, platelets, and all the other good things that will keep Eric strong and healthy. Also, prayers that Alan can get here safely on Tuesday, regardless of the predicted Minnesota snowstorm, and prayers that John, Will and Tony will get here safely next weekend, and Eric will be feeling really good when they land.

I know that your prayers, Eric's strong will, and God's goodness will see us through the next few days, and the next CaringBridge journal entry will be from his own hand. :)

Hugs all around!

Love, Mom

Favorite Comments

Like the impending Minnesota winter you both are in our prayers all of the time. We will just have to turn up the volume. Michelle we are humbled by the multiple roles of MOM #1, caregiver, nurse (which is always there, you can't differentiate when you are and aren't a nurse) and "We are here to kick cancer" health coach. I ran across a saying the other day and thought of you both: Cowboy boots may be cute, but sometimes you have to use the pointy ends, which I know you are doing!!

—Cindy Goldenstein, November 9, 2014

When you are going through Hell... Keep going. There is a light ahead.

Straight to it. Always keep faith. There are more people pulling for you and your son than you even know...
Peace.
—Mark Foss, November 8, 2014

Mom and Eric, as a mom of a cancer child, it is tough to watch, but you're on the right path. Stay ahead of the pain. I know I was so worried about Ashley getting hooked on pain killers, but they are needed. Prayers are coming. Eric's feisty. He can do this! Mom... hang in there!
—Barb Abernethy, November 8, 2014

11-10-2014: A Sweet Request

by ERIC'S MOM, Monday, November 10, 2014

Hi again, everyone!

I know you are waiting to hear from Eric, but that most likely won't happen for another day or two. And so I wanted to share a wonderful update with you: Just a short time ago Eric came down and asked for pancakes. This is super wonderful because, 1) He came out of his room, 2) He actually requested a food item rather than me going down lists and lists of food choices hoping he will choose one, and 3) Eric chose something sweet! He is sweet averse during chemo and after, and he only enjoys sweet when he is in recovery! I was so happy to get cooking and even though the pancake mix was "complete," I added an egg and milk for some hidden protein. :) I decided not to take the time for my pancake art because I did not know how much time I had til he collapsed, but he knows there is love in every bite. The exercise and meal completely wiped him out, and I don't expect to see him again until tomorrow, but, oh, I have a joyous heart right now!

To top it off, his pain is in great control. Mondays and Tuesdays are the most painful time, and he reports he's feeling pretty good: a 3 out of 10, for the nurses and doctors out there. :)

I wanted to thank you for your prayers, and just wanted you to know that they are being answered... "sweetly" answered.

Hugs all around!

Love, Mom

Favorite Comments

Good news, maybe pancakes are the answer. Leg hairs are probably not popular in California. But you need them in Minnesota to keep warm.
—Don Yetzer, November 11, 2014

I am so awed and inspired by your dedication in this journey, Michelle, and by Eric's "fight" and humor. Together you are muscling through! What a precious time for you–no, not easy, but precious and strengthening!
—Carrie Harpell, November 11, 2014

I want to be able to say something witty or really uplifting but truly the first words that come to mind are, "Michelle, I love you. Because I love you, I love your whole family." I am in awe of this journey that you all are on and the strength and humor that you share with us. Love and prayers, love, love, love...
—Kristin Ritter, November 10, 2014

11-12-2014: Oh, Hi

by ERIC GLYNN, Wednesday, November 12, 2014

I'mmmmm... back.

Whew, that was bad. But over the last couple of days I was finally able to read mom's posts, the comments, and when I finally looked at my phone and saw 40 emails and texts, I was like oh, crap, you all think I passed away.

Well here's an update: I'M ALIVE! ^_^

I actually hated most of what I read in the last couple of posts because, yeah, that all happened. Even starting Tuesday, my second day of treatment, the "blackout-feelings" and blood pressure stuff had started. But yes, my mom put it all pretty eloquently. It was a pretty sick week that I wouldn't have survived if she wasn't there to tell me it was time to get the eff up and go back to the hospital, make me eggs, bring me Cap'n Crunch and Crunch Berries.

You're doing a perfect job, mom.

I officially hate the hospital. The smells (which I will not get into), the sound of the fluid machine pumping, me feeling so full at the end of the day from the liters upon liters of hydration, steroids, anti-nausea fluids and chemo pumped into me. I believe it was Friday that there was a woman clear across the hospital just writhing and moaning in pain from what we think was some type of bone cancer. I'm assuming what she was going through was 100 times worse than the bone pain I get from my Neulasta shot, but even if it was only as bad… you just feel, with literally every pulse, pain deep in your bones coursing up your back, up to your jaw and every individual bone in between.

In conclusion… don't smoke, wear sunscreen, and for God's sake, just perform preventative checks and tests and stuff yearly so you either catch something early or avoid chemo all together, because you want no part of this. Nobody here deserves this. Like even if I saw Darth Vader or Voldemort or something, I'd be like "Hey dude, are you doing a couple prostate checks a year? Cuz that stuff can creep up on you, man…"

End fussy, stern talk

Feeling so much better now, but still shaky. I can tell that with each cycle I fall behind one to two days as far as my body bouncing back. I was healthy enough to forgo pain and nausea meds long enough to drive myself down to Huntington Beach to rest, relax and get some alone time before John, Tony and Will come out Friday. I'm so excited to see them. We'll sneak in a sunset or two, play some old school video games, maybe down a couple whiskeys, and just generally act like the four dumbasses we are when we're together.

I'll drop them off at the airport Sunday night, will have a blood results meeting at USC on Tuesday, and then that next weekend brothers Bryan and Mike are flying in. Alan flew in Tuesday with no return ticket, and is making the family of five a Thanksgiving dinner that Friday night, and then the boys will stay the weekend. The only item on the docket is to see

Dumb and Dumber To, because the three of us were obsessed with the first one growing up. Aside from that we'll try some California recreational drugs, hit up a couple strip clubs and try and walk away with thousands of dollars in gambling debts. Something like that. Right Mudder?? ;)

I'll drop them off at the airport that Sunday night, and then that Monday starts Thanksgiving week and my last week of chemo, hopefully! As long as the drugs do what they have to that last week, I won't need more, but if I need more, it'll be some intense chemo something-or-other, and a possible bone marrow transplant. Let's hope it doesn't come to that.

So let's all assume best-case scenario, that my four cycles do the job. I have my final blood work and CT scan early December, come home for the holidays (something like December 21 to January 2) and then my surgery would tentatively be on January 5. Bingo bango.

I'm still imagining walking into a clinic where Vader and Voldemort are sitting in a waiting room, waiting for their prostate exam. I walk in, give them both a nod and sit in a chair between them. I'd probably ask Vader if he could get a purple lightsaber signed by Samuel L. Jackson for me, and pass Voldemort a business card for an OC nose job plastic surgeon...... I digress...

Favorite Comments

I love your positive outlook and your focus on all the new, fun days to come. Each new day is one step closer to full recovery. Stay strong! Saying prayers for you everyday.
—Teresa Dixon, November 14, 2014

Hiya buddy... yet another entertaining, thought provoking, & informative post. Hazaaa!!! Love you so much.
—Amy Glynn, November 13, 2014

Keep the faith Eric… you are doing a tremendous job in keeping your sense of humor, your optimism, and muscling through the pain. Continued prayers. ~Godspeed.
—Jill Steinhauser, November 13, 2014

Your humor carries you my friend... don't lose it! Stay the course and know that so many of us are sending you positive thoughts. Your Thunderbolt pal,
—Norma Fields, November 12, 2014

Your attitude is amazing and your writing eloquent. God has blessed you with many gifts Eric – just need to kick this cancer out of the way so you can enjoy all that He has given you.
—Annette Glynn, November 12, 2014

Instagram 11-13-14 @eric_t_glynn

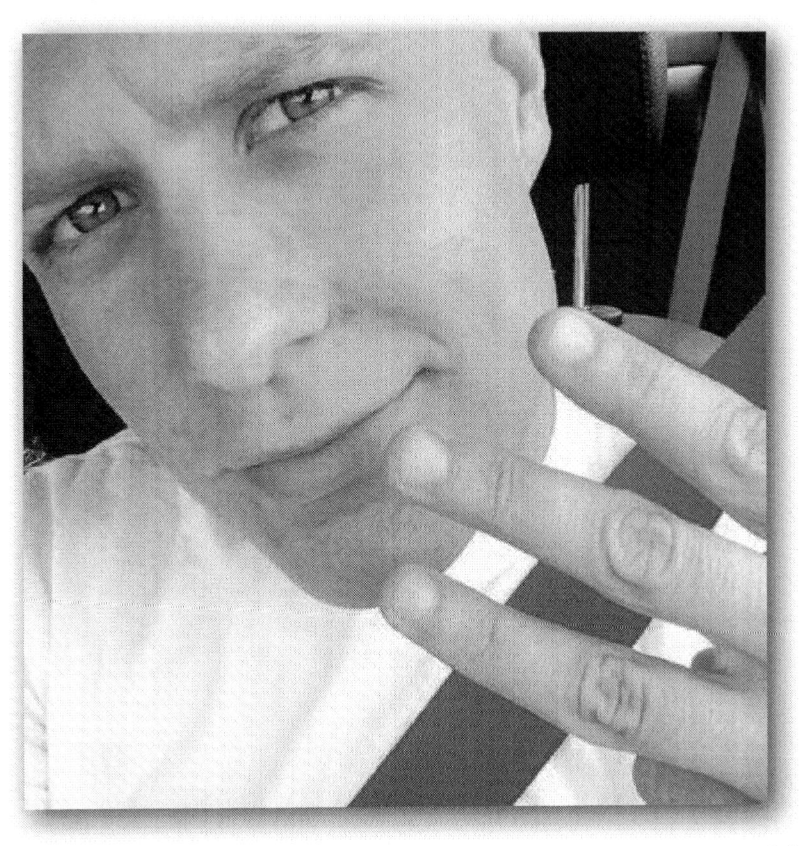

THREE chemo cycles in the bag :) One more chemo cycle to go and then hopefully chemo is DONE. A major surgery in early January and then I can finally heal up and be a normal kid again...cancer freeeeeeeeee. Your instalove continues to amaze. I adore every comment and it's been so fun to see some of you come over and read my caring bridge blogs (link in my profile). I'm fighting on for ME and for YOU. #douchyselfieoftheday #youretougherthanyouknow #fighter #cancer #chemo #support #cancersucks #instalove #loveyouguys #superbald #starttoday #fitness #workout #gym #weightlifting #fitfam #weightloss #selfie #cali #california #socal #westcoast #huntingtonbeach #hb #ca #la #losangeles

Favorite Comments

@hel*****

Congrats!!! It's such a great feeling when you only have one left to go! The day you leave the hospital after your last treatment is the best feeling! Hang in there! You got this! <3

@run*****

Your amazing will, humor and grace through everything is inspiring.

@tak*****

Your strength is amazing! Greetings from Germany, you are really special...

@the*****

You're in my prayers Eric. I can tell that you still have some valuable work to do in this world :)

@eric_t_glynn

@the***** Well said, sir.

11-16-2014: Four Baldies

by ERIC GLYNN, Sunday, November 16, 2014

Just had a great weekend with the Lakeville, Minnesota friends. Picked them up from Los Angeles International Airport (LAX) Friday afternoon, got some awesome sushi and gelato, and then played a buttload of Halo 2, our favorite game from high school, Friday night. We all sucked pretty bad. I blame my performance on the cancer… you'll have to ask the other guys what their excuses were…

Saturday we got some delicious breakfast, watched the surfers from the pier, hit a happy hour and played some pool (where we all sucked… again blaming my performance on cancer), and then hung out at my favorite hole-in-the-wall Irish bar in Huntington Beach, where we sat outside and talked with dudes who just came over on the boat from Ireland and are (illegally) living in Cali and working in landscaping. Something tells me they aren't paying taxes on said landscaping labor…

If you take a look at the pictures, you'll see that all four of us are bald right now because my friends are awesome and they shaved their heads for me. And we got a lot of funny looks from people when we'd walk down the street, or just all be chilling together at a table. We did kind of look like we were a part of a white supremacist gang, except we all dress like preppies and I'm pretty sure none of us could hurt a fly if we tried.

AWESOME to see the boys, though. Dropped them back off at LAX this morning and they are en route back home now.

As for me, bloodwork on Tuesday to see how the chemo is going, relaxing with mom and Alan in Huntington Beach all week, and then Bryan and Mike get here Friday for another good weekend.

Finally... my Movember guys are kicking ass. They're already at $745 raised, and we're only halfway through the month. If you can spare a few bucks, please make a donation! I believe you can toss in as little as $5 and any donations can be anonymous if you wish.

Mom's leg hair is growing pretty well, and Alan is rocking one hell of a salt-and-pepper beard, so both are representing Movember. I had a few facial hairs grow in, but they fell out again so… I'm trying my best here… ;)

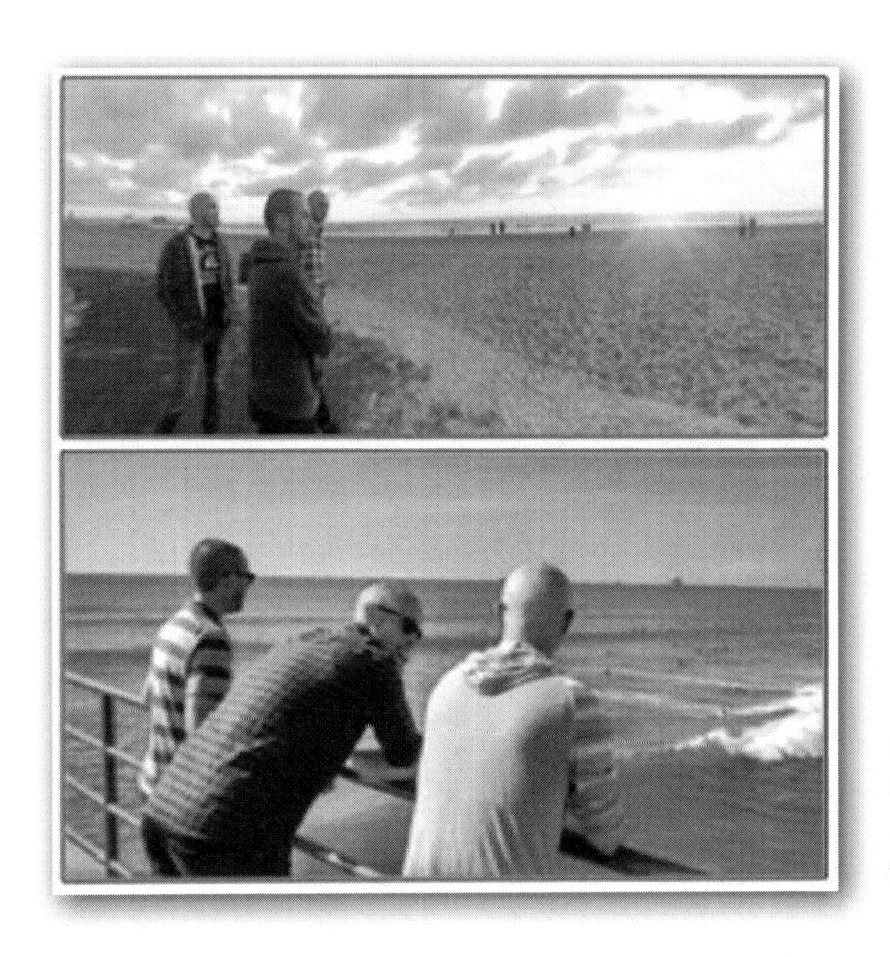

Favorite Comments

Looks like you have some competition for being Mr. Clean!
—Don Yetzer, November 17, 2014

I continue to love the posts, love your family and love the attitudes!! Keep kickin it, all!
—Kristin Ritter, November 16, 2014

One bunch of great guys!
—Patti Feldman, November 16, 2014

I'm so glad you guys had a great time! I really enjoyed your pics and your bald heads. Eric, make the most of tossing the C-card because in a few months you will have hair, you will be healed, you will be cured, and you will have to go back to relying on your dimples and personality. See you soon! Love, Mom
—Eric's mom, November 16, 2014

Instagram 11-17-14 @eric_t_glynn

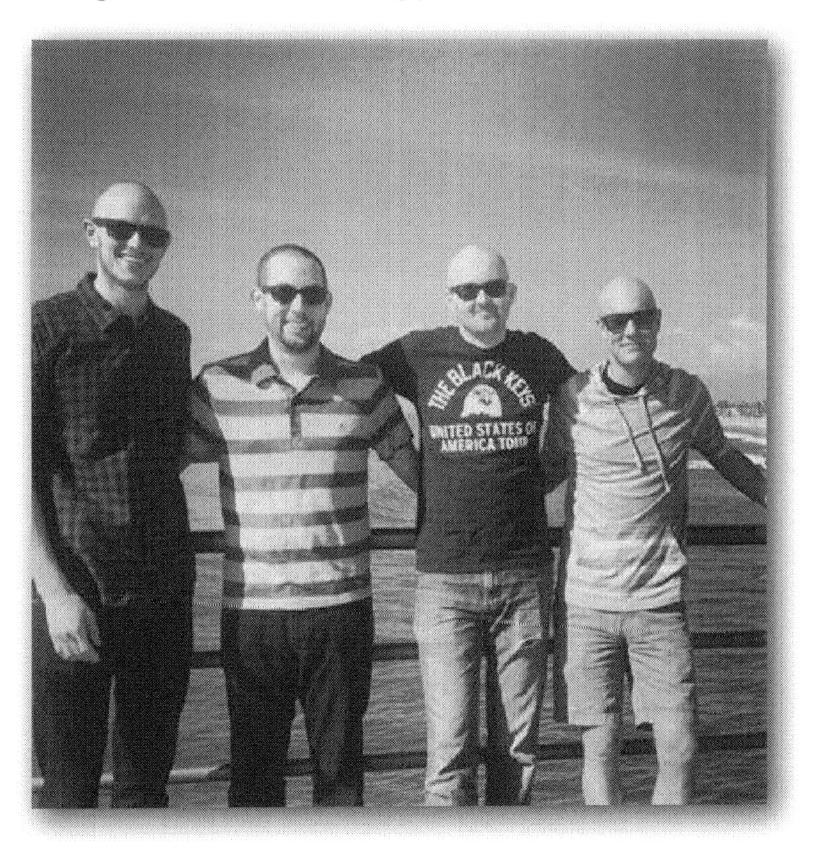

Three of my best friends from MN came to visit this weekend and they all surprised me with shaved heads as support. I have the best friends ever. Who says you can't have fun during chemo? I've also received a bunch of awesome Direct Messages this week from you all. I have the best insta friends as well ^_^ #douchyselfieoftheday #youretougherthanyouknow #fighter #cancer #chemo #support #cancersucks #instalove #loveyouguys #superbald #starttoday #fitness #workout #gym #weightlifting #fitfam #weightloss #selfie #cali #california #socal #westcoast #huntingtonbeach #hb #ca #la #losangeles

Favorite Comments

@chr***

Your friends are amazing :)

@fra***

Champs. Absolute champs!

@msj***

That's sweet of a friend... my friends are bums, I swear. Lol.

@ble***

You can always tell who your true friends are! Keep up the fight!

@law***

That's radical my friend. You give that disease some real hell aight? You got this!!!

@pun***

I find it amazing how you deal with this. My little brother had cancer when he was 2 years old (he's cancer free since 2003) so I know it really sucks. Keep your head up high and get well soon!

@len***

Awesome!! :) #bestfriends

11-18-2014: Cycle 3 Lab Results

by ERIC GLYNN, Tuesday, November 18, 2014

Hi! How are you? I have a bad cold. It sucks. My nose is running so much that I think we could somehow siphon out enough liquid from it to help solve the California drought issues. Seriously.

Today was post-cycle three blood work day:

—The AFP number should be 8.3, and I dropped from 1982 at the start to 1014 after the first cycle to 228 after the second cycle to 50.4 today.
—The HCG number should be 0.6, and I dropped from 3133 at the start to 197.2 after the first cycle to 7 after the second cycle to 1.7 today.

*A typical white blood count should be 4,000-10,900, and I have over 9,000, so we're all good and I'll be able to start cycle 4 of chemo on Monday. The doctors are confident that my HCG will be in the normal range after cycle 4, and that even if my AFP is a bit high (which it will be) after the 4th, that we'll be okay with moving forward with surgery, and just continue to monitor the number and make sure it doesn't go up, as the number should continue to drop over time (including after surgery.)

One piece that is a bit different than what I previously wrote was the surgery date. Due to the surgeon's schedule, we need to be more aggressive on the date, so for now we are scheduled for a December 22 surgery. If this is the case, I won't be making it home for the holidays, which is a bummer, but the next available surgery date after the holidays is just way too far out. And I want to get it out of the way and start healing ASAP, because even with the December 22 surgery date, I wouldn't be able to go back to work until mid-to-late March, and Eric needs to start bringing home the bacon again. Energy drinks aren't free, after all…

Favorite Comments

I am so happy your numbers are heading for health! You continue to be in my prayers for a complete recovery. Peace and power to you, Eric, as you continue to battle on.
—Vicky Menozzi, November 23, 2014

A birthday wish for your mom's December 22nd birthday... her first born son, cancer free!
—Laurie Gaikowski, November 19, 2014

Keep strong... no worries about the energy drinks... the Foss family has you covered on this! Peace buddy!
—Chris Foss, November 18, 2014

Instagram 11-23-14 @eric_t_glynn

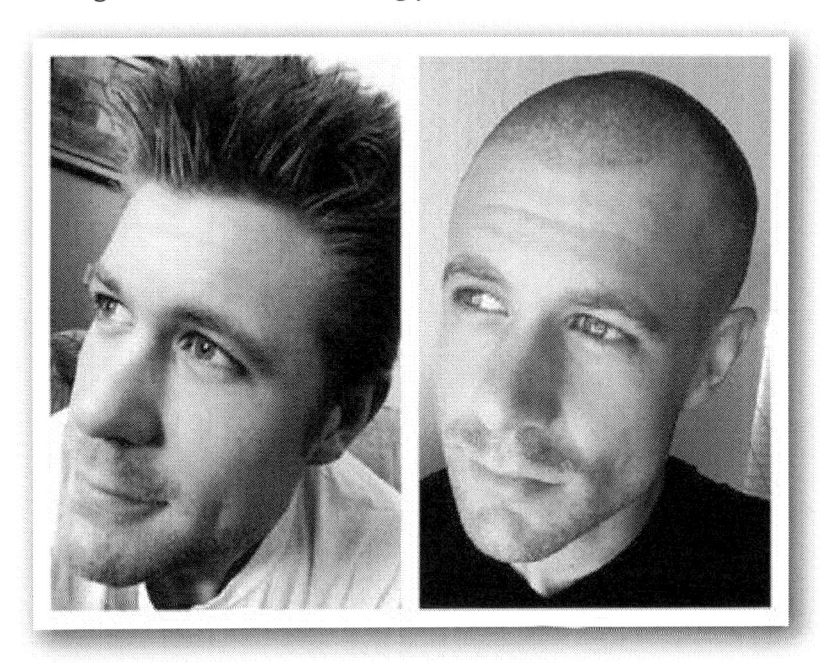

A little #tbt to when I had hair! Only a couple months ago. And then a shot right after cancer forced me into a buzzcut. But know what? I kinda like the buzzcut. Should I go back to my dishwater blonde locks after this is all over or stick with the buzzcut and 5 o'clock shadow?? #douchyselfieoftheday #youretougherthanyouknow #fighter #cancer #chemo #support #cancersucks #instalove #loveyouguys #superbald #starttoday #fitness #workout #gym #weightlifting #fitfam #weightloss #selfie #cali #california #socal #westcoast #hb #ca #la #losangeles

Favorite Comments

@ccc*****

Fight like a boss! Beat up cancer like a boxer! Make cancer the loser! Prayers for youuuu...

@ata*****

I hope everything is going really well with your treatment. My dad was diagnosed with stage 4 lymphoma in March and he has just been through chemo all year and now finished radiotherapy and everything possible... crossed all the roads to recovery. :) I wish all the same for you <3

@ale*****

I've just been humbled by your #instajourney. Thank you for that. You are amazing. And as of today, you've got one more cheerleader screaming, praying and flipping for your complete and expedient recovery. You're a blessing "Mr. Cancer."

@jam*****

Buzz cut and scruff is sexy.

@san*****

I personally think having veeery short hair makes our eyes stand out more! You look great. I have just seen all of your pics, now I know your story. I know you must have read this a thousand times, but you are a great role model. I wish I could give you a biiig hug but still... virtual hugs for you from Mexico City!!!! Hehe. Thanks for liking my pic too ;)

@kay*****

There's something about a buzz cut that instantly makes a guy hotter. I'm inspired by the fact that you see the negative as a positive as much as you can regardless of the circumstances. You are an inspiration to people fighting their own battles. #YoureSomebodysHero

@xik***

I prefer you in the second pic, with victory and experience in your eyes :)

@san***

There's something to be said about the time it saves getting ready in the morning. I just slap my wig on after a shower and I'm out the door. I like either look you have here, but know from experience you just want to see hair again. Now I'm growing chemo hair, which is the frizz curly hair. Not loving that so much :)

@kim***

I don't know about you, but I feel like such a different person, inside and out, since cancer and chemo! Good luck and happiness to you!

11-23-2014: Bro Weekend, Time For Cycle 4

by ERIC GLYNN, Sunday, November 23, 2014

Great to see the brothers this weekend. Alan treated the family of five to a Thanksgiving dinner on Friday, and then mom and Alan headed back to LA so the three of us could have bro time. We ate a ton of food (all of which was bad for our health), played some football on the beach (I lasted about four minutes before this hairless pile of skin and bones I call my current body ran out of stamina), went to *Dumb and Dumber To* (which could have been much worse), and snuggled up to a couple movies at night (award winning films, like *Jackass 2*). It was a good, typical 48 hours of Glynn bro time.

It's been a great 10 days in Huntington Beach seeing awesome people. It's actually felt like a really long time since my last cycle of chemo. Time did not fly by, even though I was having a lot of fun, which is nice. But it's time to go back to the real world. My fourth (and hopefully final) round of chemo starts tomorrow. I can't believe I have to go back to that hospital and do this again. After my final shot and fluid bag on Saturday afternoon, I'm going to give that entire day hospital a huge finger, as I really, really hope I never have to walk through those doors again.

I'm prepared for this last cycle to be the worst though, as I'm not walking into it feeling 100 percent like I did after the first two cycles. I still have a little cold, and feel like 80 percent. The cycles have definitely added up and taken a bit of a toll. Bah, won't sleep so great tonight.

I can't wait for my journal entry where I can say "I'm baaaakcckckckckckkkk" for the fourth and final time. Until then you will probably be hearing from my lovely Mudder. Here. We. Go.

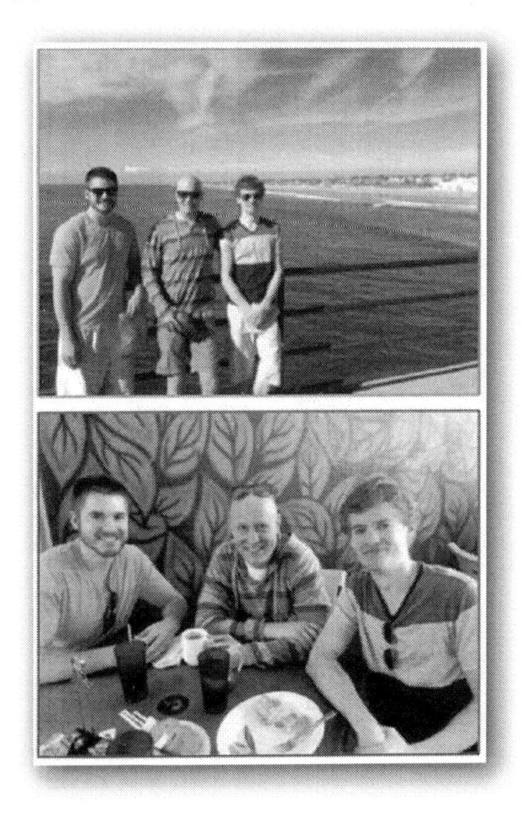

Favorite Comments

I honestly can't say I have any idea what you're going through. I'm sure it's 1000 times more brutal than I can even picture. I'm just praying that it will be nowhere near as bad as you think, and that it will definitely be the last one you'll ever have to do. I wish you strength and courage and total healing.
—Wendy H, November 24, 2014

Can't wait for your next "I'm baaaakcckckckckckkkk" entry. Thinking about you and hoping it isn't too brutal. Soon, this will all be behind you! Hugs and prayers............
—Mary Jo Jasper, November 24, 2014

You can give your chemo IV bags the finger, but I hope you will use your hands for hugs, high fives, fist bumps, and goodbye waves. USC team has been awesome from cleaning staff to volunteers to Chaplain, nurses, doctors, and the most important player: Nancy the really cool scheduler! Sleep well, my son. You are so covered with prayer you are glowing. LOVE the pics. Love, Mom
—Eric's mom, November 23, 2014

Kick ass this week Erix. One more f&%#ing cycle and you can close that s&%@#y chapter my friend.
—John Feldman, November 23, 2014

You got this, Glynn! Will definitely be thinking about you, man. It's such great news hearing you're on your last round of chemo. We continue to pray for you for strength and endurance through this whole thing. Take care of yourself and continue to kick cancer's balls!
—Sarah Johnson, November 23, 2014

One more round friend and then kiss that crap goodbye. You've rocked it this far, and you're gonna take on the last round the same way. Lots of love from me and Allison.
—Anthony Giorgi, November 23, 2014

11-27-14: GivingThanks

by ERIC'S MOM, Thursday, November 27, 2014

Happy Thanksgiving, everyone!

It's been a weird Thanksgiving. I asked Eric what he was thankful for today and he replied, "Silence." Hmmmm… this was going to be a hard day for me… I asked Alan, and he said he was thankful to be here with Eric and I. Me… ? I am so thankful for the ongoing love and support and encouragement and prayers of family, friends, and friends I have not met yet, and for technology like this where my fingers can do the talking so that Eric can enjoy silence. :)

It's been a weird chemo day. Eric has been going to the outpatient chemo clinic at USC, and has the same chemo nurse almost every time (and we LOVE her!), but because of the holiday, outpatient chemo was closed, so Eric had to spend the day in the cancer hospital to stay on track with his chemo cycle. Though his nurse was very nice and also quite cute, they are not used to regimes like Eric's, so things ran a bit slower. And though chemo is killing Eric's patience, along with his cancer cells, he drank the chemo when the nurse wasn't looking just to speed things up a bit. Eric's hospital Thanksgiving lunch was sent up, so Alan and I went down to the cafeteria and enjoyed a truly fabulous turkey dinner… honestly, it was awesome! When we got back to the room, we asked Eric how his Thanksgiving meal was. Well, it was one of those "guess the meat" deals. And the correct answer: un-named fish. So, Alan and I went back to the cafeteria and got Eric a turkey dinner.

Gobble, gobble.

Eric has done pretty well this fourth and final chemo cycle. They have been giving him more IV fluid hydration the last few days, and it was helpful at first, but he is getting more dizzy and nauseated with each day, and still having issues of very low blood pressure when he stands. Tomorrow is the last day of chemo, praise the Lord!

Some good news to report: One of Eric's cancer markers, HCG, was at 0.9 on Monday, so it is nearly at the undetectable range! Woot! The AFP, however, is being very stubborn, but hopefully this cycle, my homemade chicken soup, and your prayers will take care of that.

Hugs all around! Enjoy your holiday weekend! Safe travels, all!

Eric, just one more day of chemo! Never to return except to show off your new hair to the nurses! You got this, son!

Love, Mom

Favorite Comments

Eric. The end is getting closer. Hopefully you have now been through the worst part. Isn't it amazing how strong your spirit can be… even when you feel you can't go on another day? So proud of you… I look forward to your posts as you always put a smile on my face. As a mother of boys, I get your humor and actually get a laugh… (that seems pretty bad that I am

laughing at the cancer kid, but you are quite funny!) I'm also praying and sending my best healing thoughts. You are an amazing person and I have a feeling God is working through you in ways you don't even know yet! Michelle, I now know where Eric got his gift of the written word and getting those words on paper in such a profound way. My mother's heart has broken with yours, but also laughed at your humor in dealing with grown "men children." You are one STRONG lady who has been forced to deal with a mother's greatest worry. I send hugs, love, and prayers for continued strength and peace.
—Jill Zweber, December 1, 2014

Michelle, you make me smile every time you post! I can hear your voice and your laugh. Covering all of you in prayer and looking forward to seeing Eric with a beautiful head of hair again! Although, he is so cute with or without hair!
—Laurie Gaikowski, November 28, 2014

12-2-2014: No Mo' Chemo :)

by ERIC GLYNN, Tuesday, December 2, 2014

I'm back. :D :D :D :D

Seriously, eff that chemo stuff. Thank you for killing cancer and all, but let's go our separate ways. It's truly for the best. Don't try and call me 'cuz I'm gonna block your number.

This cycle was weird. Mom, Alan and I spent Thanksgiving in the hospital. I was laying there that day thinking about everyone in Minnesota all dressed in your winter sweaters, fireplaces on, football on, drinking beer while the smells of Thanksgiving filled whatever house you were inside. Meanwhile, I was being served this yellowish, wrinkled up blob they called "fish," in a plastic tray. You seriously should have seen it. Mom was all excited about the turkey dinner they were serving in the cafeteria, and the nurse said they'd send one up to me. And then that pile of garbage showed up. It was a predictable, if not an imperfectly appropriate ending to one awesome day.

By Friday, I was just over it. I couldn't just lie in bed and wait for the day to be over with my eyes closed like normal. I was pacing around the room (well, I guess "pacing" means sitting up and laying down again because it's sort of hard to pace when you're both in a 9 ft x 9 ft room and you're plugged into IV machines.) But we got through the day, got through the hydration day on Saturday, and I've just been resting up at home since.

I haven't exactly been 100 percent knocked out these last four days like I usually am after a week of chemo. Kind of in-and-out. Super, super tired. After a meal I have to lie down again. Walked to Subway today, and needed a nap when I got home. Like, pathetically weak. But I think we have the pain meds, the nausea meds… pretty much every med known to man down pat, to where we know when and how to take them and it helps. Also, I think the psychology of knowing that this almost certainly is my last cycle of chemo is helping with me just wanting to be over and past it… to fast forward to the part where I just rest for a few weeks.

So, these next few weeks…

Next Tuesday, December 9, we will be doing blood work and an updated CT scan. Hopefully the blood work shows that the levels are okay enough for surgery, and the CT scan will show us our first physical images of my lymph node tumor since before chemo started. A miracle would show that it's so small that it doesn't need to even be operated on, but realistically it will show that it is SAFE ENOUGH to be operated on, and then we'd lock in the December 22 surgery date for sure. I believe the 16th is our surgical consult date to go over everything.

So, I basically have 20 days of rest between now and the surgery date, and I'll need every day. No out of town visitors planned, no big events. Just resting and building up strength for this last phase. The surgery is called "Retroperitoneal Lymph Node Dissection," I believe. Give that a Google search if you're interested to learn more or just… like gore. Blech. I'll explain it more after our surgical consult.

One quick update. Movember is over! My Movember boys ended up raising $1,145, so they exceeded their $1,000 goal! Good job, boys.

Time to pack and then head to Huntington Beach tonight. It'll be a great place to rest these next few weeks. I'm pretty drugged up so I probably won't be doing the driving. Actually, I probably shouldn't be typing in this condition. Did any of that stuff make sense up there? Can anybody hear me?

Favorite Comments

Loud and clear, bub. Loud and clear.
—Mark Foss, December 3, 2014

Good job buddy, keep on trucking, looking forward to blowing off some steam soon.
—Mark Harrison – HB Buddy, December 2, 2014

So I had everything planned for a safe cycle 4 for Eric: Alan is here as a second body for driving, parking, running errands and providing strong arms and shoulders for both Eric and me as needed. And our hosts provided us with a wheelchair, as I was certain Eric was not going to safely navigate car to chemo on days 4, 5 and 6 this round since we nearly lost him a few times in cycle 3. But though his blood pressure got as low as 75/36 (yikes) the kid took this round stronger than any of the other cycles! Last cycle he did not shower from Wednesday to Wednesday, but this time he was showering nearly everyday, had cravings for pizza and chicken alfredo, and was feeling good enough to be "bored." He only asked for a gun once, and that was on Thursday. He considered watching football, but decided against it in the end. I was starting to worry that the pharm tech forgot to put the chemo into the IV bags! :) Eric was doing so well that Alan and I left him on Sunday to go on a date to one of Mario Batali's LA restaurants, courtesy of a gift card from Eric's friends to us when they were here to visit. Thanks, men! We brought food home for Eric as well.

I am SO happy Eric has done so well this cycle! Eric, I have never been prouder of you :) You deserve this break! Love, Mom

—Eric's mom, December 2, 2014

Eric, the end is near! You have been a trooper through this entire ordeal. We continue to send prayers your way. Get the rest you need so you have the strength for surgery.

—Shelly O'Brien, December 2, 2014

Good work, Eric. Let me know if you need a nap partner; I'll support you by napping with you over Skype. I hope it never happens, but if I ever have some sort of extended disease treatment, I can only hope I'll deal with it as well as you have been.
—Brandon, December 2, 2014

The nurse in me had to Google it. Can I scrub in on your surgery? I'll just be the circulator. I promise I won't stick my arm in your abdomen. :) I've been the circulator for C-sections... that's almost the same right?
—Kristy Maguire, December 2, 2014

Instagram 12-5-14 @eric_t_glynn

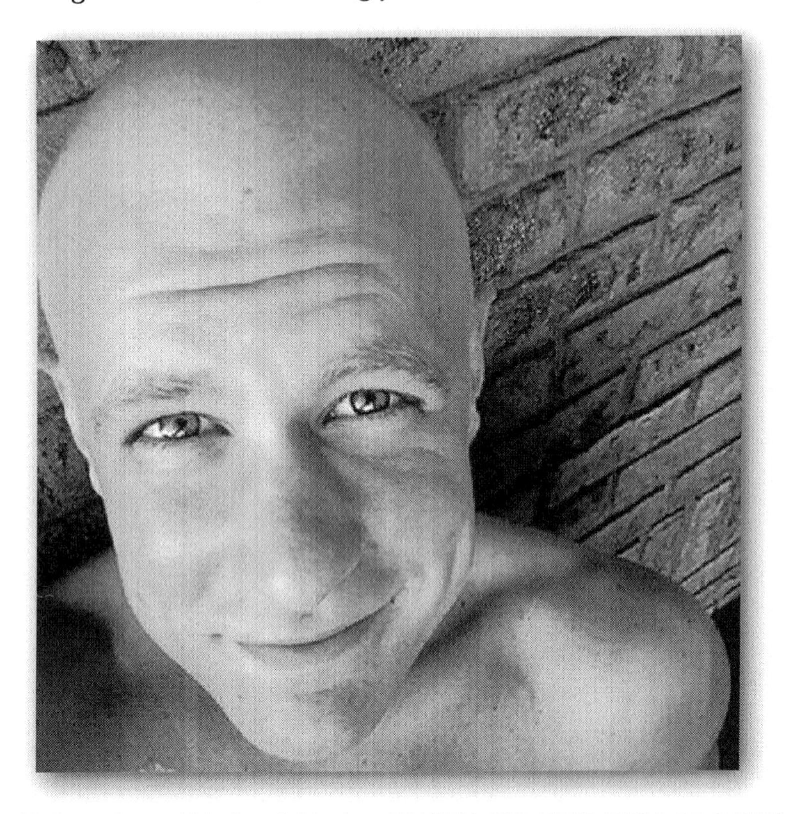

This is one happy kid. I just finished my FOURTH AND FINAL CYCLE OF CHEMO. I now get to rest up in Huntington Beach for a few weeks and then a major surgery on December 22 to get rid of the rest of the cancer and officially put it in remission. Thank you so much for all the kind words, encouragement and stories over this whole time. I read every comment and it's been great interacting with you in the comments section. I'm almost through this, guys...thanks for fighting with me. #douchyselfieoftheday #youretougherthanyouknow #fighter #cancer #chemo #support #cancersucks #instalove #loveyouguys #superbald #starttoday #fitness #workout #gym #weightlifting #fitfam #weightloss #selfie #cali #california #socal #westcoast #huntingtonbeach #hb #ca #la #losangeles

Favorite Comments

@kco*****

Well done, you. I've spent the last few years surrounded by cancer so it fills my heart to hear such positivity. XO

@sun*****

Crossing my fingers and everything else that your world contains only happiness, laughter and all other good stuff for you.

@sfd*****

Hang in there Eric! I have fought stage 4 metastatic melanoma twice now so if I can beat it, so can you. It's all about the attitude. Accept nothing but total victory.

@amr*****

Keep it up, man... hope you heal fast... cheers from Egypt! :)

@mis*****

Stay strong!!! I also have cancer, but it's brain cancer and it hurts. But life must go on! Keep calm, I'm with you <3

@car*****

Your soul can be seen through your eyes <3 My youngest cousin has been struggling with breast cancer for more than a year now and she is as brave as you. You guys are real inspirations!!! Hope you have good news.

@tam***

It's the first day I've heard of you. I came across you when you liked my pic and I went through your gallery and automatically I could see that you've been through so much. I love your gallery and I really admire you for being such a strong human being. Being able to fight through chemo and have them work on your body takes a lot. It takes a #REAL man to overlook all obstacles. You're such a positive influence to many.

@ohm***

Wow. I'm blown away by your story. So inspiring!!! Keep sharing... you're showing the world what's really possible!

@ral***

I truly believe that the eyes are the gateway to the soul – and what a beautiful and mischievous soul I see!

@rib***

You're an inspiration! I lost my dad in May '14 and now my mom... well they say she has six months. She is 78 and just doesn't have it in her to fight. It's nice to see the flip side in your journey of someone that will. Please always keep fighting!! Never give up your positive vibe, it helps more than you know.

12-9-2014: Surgery Is A GO

by ERIC GLYNN, Tuesday, December 9, 2014

So mom and I just got back from the hospital appointments an hour ago.

We did blood work and got great news. The HCG number should be 0.6 and my number is... 0.6! So bingo bango bongo there. And my AFP number should be 8.3, and it's sitting at 11.7, so we're just off there. We'll be doing more blood work the next two weeks so we should see it continue to fall a bit. Even if it does end up one or two points higher than the 8.3 normal, we'll be fine and we'll just have to monitor it.

We also did a CT scan to see how the tumor looks. As predicted, the tumor has shrunk by more than half the original size, and is at a size that we can operate on.

So it is official! Surgery is on the books for December 22. Mom and I will go to the preoperative visit next Tuesday, where we'll learn all about the procedure and the post-op healing schedule and then that following Monday is the surgery date. Much like Thanksgiving, I'll be in a hospital bed for Christmas... but that's by choice. I could have stalled on the surgery for a couple more weeks, but I just want to start healing so everyyyything gggg will be behind me sooner.

One bummer is that this conflicts with the stand-up comedy date that Elysse's friend had offered to me. But it's ok. In thinking about it all, I think I could do a lot more good writing a book over doing comedy. Maybe I'd want to do something like that sometime in the future, but I dunno. Would be fun, but as I'm getting deeper and deeper into this whole cancer world, I'm getting into a mode where I'd rather help people going through it, over risking the chance of offending people who have been touched by cancer. I guess I'm turning into a softie.

So that's kinda it. I've been a lazy bum the last week, watching "The Voice" and "The Office" with mom, sleeping in late… and that's what I plan to do these next 13 days before surgery too. I dunno how I'll ever go back to setting an alarm and getting up for work. Eff that.

Oh! I also had a pulmonary function test today, which tests your lung capacity and strength and stuff, and all my results were over 100 percent of the expected value for my age and sex. One of the tests I got like 240 percent. So, like, next time there's a forest fire in California, just bring me in and I should blow it out with one gust.

A fireman… that's what I'll be when this is all over. It's all coming together now.

Favorite Comments

What better Christmas gift than to have that tumor GOOOONE!!!! So glad you're doing well. We're pulling for you! You inspire me every day. Will be good to read about your journey in your book. Best wishes from one of your fans!! Mwah!! HB
—Helen Blythe-Hart, December 15, 2014

It IS all coming together. Never thought of any other possibility. Straight ahead, Eric.
You got this.
—Mark Foss, December 13, 2014

Hi Eric, so glad you got the news we were all hoping for! Enjoy the time off and get your rest for surgery. It's too bad you will be spending Christmas in the hospital, but you will brighten everyone else's holiday in there with you. We continue to send love and prayers.
—Shelly O'Brien, December 10, 2014

So excited to read your post. We are so happy for you and your family... I don't blame you for wanting it all behind you and spending Christmas in the hospital... I hope you spread good Christmas cheer to the others in there. You can be their blessing this year... prayers for you as your prepare for surgery and for the surgery to be a complete success!!!
—Dan and Trish Dysthe, December 10, 2014

So glad to see you at church with your mom, Eric! Hope we didn't freak you out by praying over you like that! But we'll keep praying until C has had its butt kicked and has run off squealing. ;-)
—Wendy H, December 10, 2014

I like seeing the progression of how your posts have become more and more medical sounding. I think all that time around hospitals has rubbed off on you.
—Scott Deeney, December 9, 2014

Can you hear all of your Minnesota fans screaming from where you are???? Great news, Eric! I hope your mom is taking advantage of the great wine out there. :) Stay strong!
—Kristin Ritter, December 9, 2014

You are sooo dang funny! Yup, the next forest fire in CA... you're the man! :) (Made me laugh out loud sitting here by myself!) Glad you have new clarity on your future. :) I think of you & your special mom often.
—Pam Kuhr, December 9, 2014

Instagram 12-12-14 @eric_t_glynn

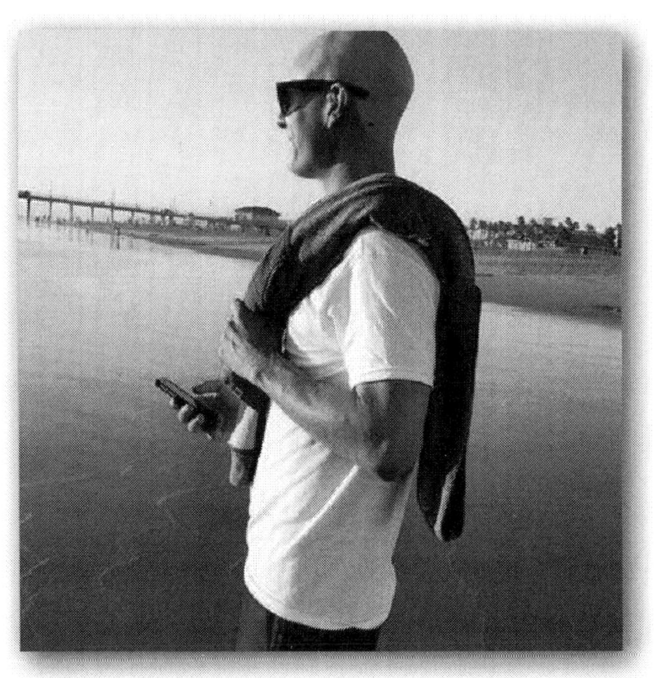

Still just resting up for surgery and dipping my foot in the ocean a lil bit :) I'M INTERESTED IN WRITING A MEMOIR about this whole battle, using my blogs, personal journals and Instagram photos and messages...yes, your messages may show up in my book! I want to give hope to the hopeless and show how important a positive attitude is during tough times. I'M WONDERING IF ANYONE IS OR KNOWS A PUBLISHER or anyone in the book writing/publishing/agency field who could help me out? If so please leave a comment or send me a Direct Message. Or feel free to share the blog that is in my profile...I want to get the word out any way I can! Thanks so much for the continued support my Instafriends!! #douchyselfieoftheday #youretougherthanyouknow #fighter #cancer #chemo #support #cancersucks #instalove #loveyouguys #superbald #starttoday #fitness #workout #gym #weightlifting #fitfam #weightloss #selfie #cali #california #socal #westcoast #huntingtonbeach #hb #ca #la #losangeles

Favorite Comments

@cha***

That's a great idea. There isn't enough sharing of positive experiences in life, let alone something as inspirational as your story. Truthfully, I would recommend looking into self-publishing: cut out the middle-man for the moment. You have tons of friends and followers who would support you and share with their crowds. It'll be a good gauge to see where things can go without the pressure of a publishing company breathing down your neck and counting copies sold/ downloaded. Something to consider.

@pau***

I really hope you get to publish your book!! Good luck with that, blessings! :)

@kgr***

Your story continues to draw me in. The humor, the strength, the silliness, acceptance. You are an amazing man. With an awesome attitude! The world needs more positive outlooks. For yours I wanna say thank you.

@vdd***

You're very inspiring. Stay strong and keep that great attitude. I just started to read some of your blog and think your book would be very encouraging. There are people fighting all kinds of battles that can benefit.

@tot***

My granddad died from cancer recently. We used to be so close and we kinda drifted away. I didn't see him in like 2 years and was planning to go and see him but it didn't happen in time. Please beat cancer's butt, for yourself and for others who need hope for their families who may be battling cancer xxxxxx you are beautiful xxxxxx

@kim***
You're living life correctly, sir. And I've found myself very fond of you and quite actually shed a couple tears seeing what you've been through and how you're taking it. Thank you for sharing and being amazing... from what I see... all around. :) Smile.

@dra***
Amazing! Thank you for sharing and being authentic! Means a lot! Sending light!

@its***
I absolutely love the idea of your writing a memoir! I've only just found your IG but, honestly, you're such an inspiration. You're strong and I know you'll get through this. Best wishes xx

12-17-2014: Some Surgery Specifics

by ERIC GLYNN, Wednesday, December 17, 2014

Five days until a surgeon cuts me open and goofs around inside my stomach! Neat...

Mom and I met with my surgeon today. The appointment was scheduled for 1 p.m.... cut to 5 p.m., and we're still in the waiting room. It was great. Truly. Great. Effffffffff. But thanks to some work by Elysse, our lovely case manager, we FINALLY got in to see him around 5:15 p.m.

We have ourselves one confident surgeon, Dr. Sia Daneshmand. The dude drives a Ferrari, speaks on surgeon panels all over the world, and told us that the surgery will go great. No real surprises on the surgery piece, really. He'll cut me from my chest bone past my belly button. He's extra fancy in that his procedure doesn't really disrupt my intestines and bowels and stuff much, so if all goes to plan it should be a 3-day hospital stay post-surgery, and I should be eating solid foods again 1-2 days after surgery. Even though the tumor is just on one side, he's going to remove the lymph nodes on both sides... just clear them all out. And if he can, he'll be able to leave my left kidney alone unless the tumor is just too wrapped around it... then he'll just pull that kidney out.

No cardio for six weeks, no lifting weights for eight weeks after surgery, which is the lame part for me. I was a fitness freak up until I got diagnosed in September, so it's been really tough to see my body deteriorate and my stamina go way down. I tried doing a typical workout that I normally did on a "light" workout day. Usually I'd do three sets of 30 push-ups, five minutes of planks and 400-800 calories burned on the elliptical, as a "rest day" between heavy weight lifting days. Yesterday's glorious stats: 12 TOTAL push-ups, one 30 second plank, and I thought I was going to throw up after 100 calories burned on the elliptical. It's funny, but also sad and sucky how fast stamina and strength can drop when you're just sitting on your ass and drinking chemo for three months.

So now I'm flying solo in Huntington Beach for five more days and mom is up in LA. Alan will fly in this weekend, and then I'll head up Sunday night as we have to arrive at the hospital at 5 a.m. on Monday for surgery prep. I'll be switching over to long-term disability, get terminated by my company and have some other odds and ends to wrap up before the surgery happens, so I'll stay busy.

I'm sure you'll get a post or two from mom over the next week while I'm under the knife and all drugged up and recovering. Should I not make it through this, I'd like to officially will my car, Ruby, to my mother. She can also have my blow-up mattress because I know she loves it. Dad and Mary can have my Von Hayes rookie card (inside joke), and my brothers can split my video games and the rest of my baseball card collection. I'll donate everything else to charity. And donate my brain to science, because someone so weird should get analyzed. The first person to copy and paste my blog entries into a Microsoft Word document gets the rights to my biography.

Just kidding. I have literally no worries going into this. I just want it done so the healing can begin. Think about me a little bit on Monday if you remember, and I'll be back soon!

Favorite Comments

Hey Eric- Keep your eye on the prize! Push-ups and planks will be back in your daily routine soon, though for some of us, we can't imagine wanting to do either of those things by choice. It's great to hear you have such a gifted surgeon. Your great attitude helps us know you're in good hands. Good luck on Monday and getting back home ASAP- We will be praying for you. Take care!
—Sue Ellen Olson, December 19, 2014

I ALWAYS love reading your posts, Eric and I was with you until the last paragraph. I'm a mom so as far as bequeathing your treasures, I will just tell you now to shut your pie hole, kiddo. I can do that because I am now 50. Yeaaaa for a rock star surgeon, yeaaaaaa for a rock star family and waaaaaay yeaaaaaa for someone who can do 12 more push-ups than a lot of teenagers and can also define what a "plank" is to them. You are a winner and I am proud to share your journey with people who need to find strength like yours. Blessings and healing prayers continued your way.
—Kristin Ritter, December 17, 2014

Dodged a big one there. Thought you were going to will me your hair gel collection. BIG relief here. Good luck man. I'm still not going to take it easy on you in our sh*tty fantasy football matchup.
—David Slifka, December 17, 2014

Keep those spirits high, Eric. You'll be planking–whatever the hell that is–again in no time.
—MarkRisa Palony, December 17, 2014

Instagram 12-19-14 @eric_t_glynn

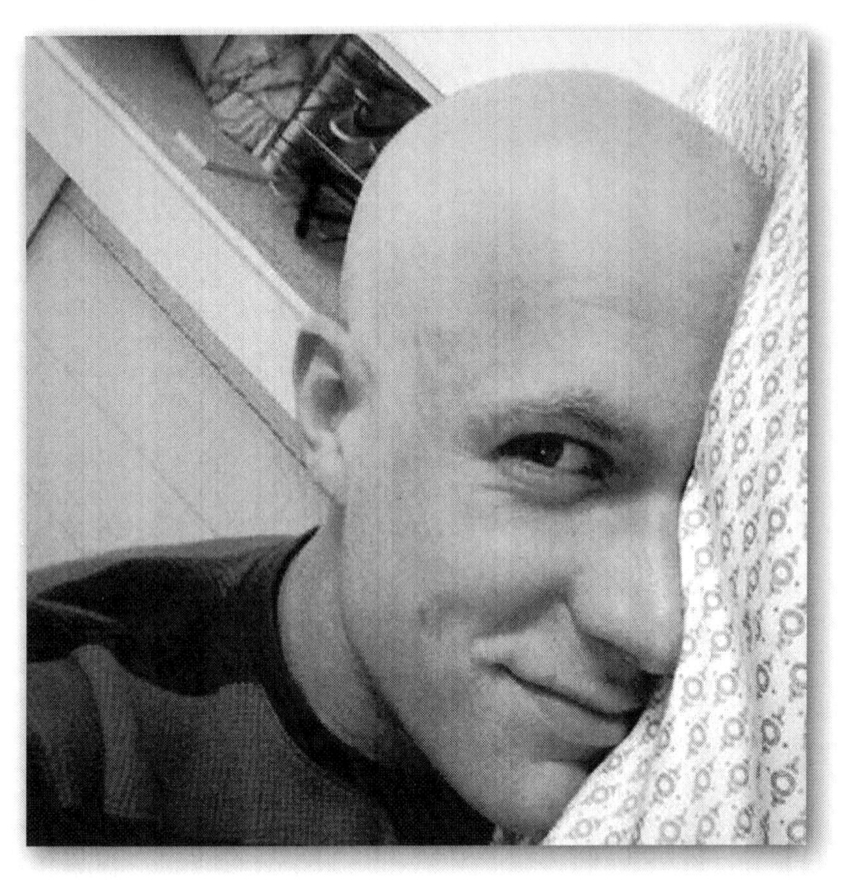

Surgery in 3 days! I should officially be in remission by the end of the day on Monday :) You can't see it but I have a liiiiiiittle bit of peach fuzz growing on my head. Cmon hair, you can do it! #douchyselfieoftheday #youretougherthanyouknow #fighter #cancer #chemo #support #cancersucks #instalove #loveyouguys #superbald #starttoday #fitness #workout #gym #weightlifting #fitfam #weightloss #selfie #cali #california #socal #westcoast #huntingtonbeach #hb #ca #la #losangeles

Favorite Comments

@mvo******

I wish you the very best of luck! Big hugs from Brazil <3

@pau***

Good luck on surgery!! You can do this!! We are all with you!

@mar***

You're so strong and amazing, Eric! <3

@cau***

You remind me so much of a dear friend of mine that I sadly lost. He never stopped smiling! Sadly for him there was never a chance of a good outcome but he was strong and caring and happy! Stay strong and keep smiling! Sending you positive thoughts. XO

@bri***

You're my favorite person.

@bri***

I want to be friends with you.

@bri***

Your eye color is rad.

@sha***

That is awesome! Wishing you the best! My man is in remission also! He also fought the fight and kicked cancer's ass. You can too! Just keep thinking positive.

@nad***

You're an amazing man. I cried when I saw and read your IG and blog. Have a great day.

@hey***

So I was looking through your journey and I know you've heard this before, but you're an amazing person with an amazing story! You're doing better than great and I hope you do go into infinite remission!

@cra***

YOU CAN DO IT (in a Rob Schneider voice)

@sha***

2015 is your year! Claim it! The universe is listening! Congrats! #inspirational

@bbr***

I had to comment on this because, for one, you're adorable and for two, you have my bed sheets lol. Being a nurse this caught my eye. I just browsed your entire page #noshame and wanted to say keep your beautiful head up. :) Cheers to your inspiring journey from getting healthy to kicking cancer's ass. So looking forward to your transformation post-cancer. I know it's gonna be great.

12-22-2014: Surgery Complete!

By ERIC'S MOM, Monday, December 22, 2014

Hi!

Great news to share! Eric's surgery went super well and only took four hours. The surgeon was able to remove the entire tumor and spare Eric's kidney. They were also able to spare his nerves. The surgeon was super happy with how things went and how things looked, and though we have to wait one to two weeks for the final pathology report, the team is pretty sure what was left behind is benign. Pray Out Loud! (POL)

Eric is settled into his room on the sixth floor. He is obviously a celebrity, as he has a corner room with a view of white-capped mountains and the rising sun. He has some great pain control going on, and he can already start with sips and ice chips. I think some hair grew back while he was on the table, his voice is deeper and he wants to go home. :)

Thank you all so very, very much for your prayers and encouragement and support! Prayers have been answered since before the diagnosis even occurred, and it is because we are surrounded by so many wonderful family and friends and friends-we-haven't-met, a spectacular health team, and an awesome God.

Hugs all around!

Love, Mom

Favorite Comments

So happy to hear this great news. God is so great. Fought through the storm to get to the other side... way to conquer Eric! Merry Christmas!
—Jill Zweber, December 24, 2014

Great job kicking that cancer in the balls. The news is a great Christmas gift for all of us that are praying & rooting for you! Miss you. Have a Merry Christmas!

—Greg Yetzer, December 23, 2014

Awesome news, not surprised though since Erix is a badass! Super happy everything went well!
—John, December 22, 2014

So happy to hear how well the surgery went! Eric must be ecstatic to have the surgery behind him and just concentrate on healing. He is one tough guy, with a remarkable mother!
—Patti Feldman, December 22, 2014

That is wonderful news!! Praise God for Eric's amazing attitude and doctors!! I hope you can all sleep tonight!! Thank you so much for the update!! Xoxoxo
—Kathleen Cassidy Duffey, December 22, 2014

Eric, praise God! He did it again. Now all the tough stuff is over and the real healing begins – healing of body (of course), healing of spirit (how you think) and healing from doubt into perfect alignment with God's plan for your future. This has just been a test and now you will be all the stronger for it. Wow, heavy stuff but let's just revel in it!!!
Ciao with love,
—Anna Glynn aka Gramma, December 22, 2014

That's amazing!!! We are so happy – Eric deserves to be finished with this crazy business and get on with his wonderful life. Much love to you, Michelle :)
—Teresa Borszcz, December 22, 2014

12-24-2014: "Jingle Balls, Jingle Balls..."

by ERIC'S MOM, Wednesday, December 24, 2014

If you think about it, there are a lot of holiday songs that with one tweak of a vowel, or a few letters, and you have a perfect celebration song for cured testicular cancer. :)

Just wanted to give everyone an update on how Eric is doing. First of all, all he is asking of Santa this year is for discharge orders, and we are hopeful those will come tomorrow. The biggest issue has been pain control. Eric was having tons of itching from the pain medication in his epidural, so it has kept him from comfort and sleep. Benadryl did not help, and stopping the narcotic portion of the epidural did not help, so he was started on orals yesterday, and this morning they turned off the epidural with hopes to remove it and his catheter by the end of today, or tomorrow morning, at the latest. They are ordering an abdominal binder to see if that helps support him better during walks, getting out of bed, etc. As soon as bowel, bladder and pain are all successfully managed, he will get to discharge. He is drinking well, and eating regular foods well, but would someone please deliver a Dominos pizza and slip in a Diet Coke with Jameson, and a lime?

Alan and I spent the morning with him, and will return to-night to sing Christmas carols over him and watch our home church's service online. Eric will be too weak to kick us out, so unless he calls security, we will have a blessed Christmas Eve "church" together in his hospital room. :)

I hope this message finds all of you where you most want to be for Christmas, surrounded by friends and family, and feeling healthy and strong, singing joyfully, and celebrating Christmas in all it's awe and wonder.

Merry Christmas!!! Hugs all around!

Love, Mom

Favorite Comments

Keeping the Jameson in the freezer (don't laugh, it works...) for when the kid gets on his feet. Ya'll come by anytime. Merry Christmas Eric, mom and all the family. Deck those Halls! (Just couldn't pull the trigger on that one...)
—Mark Foss, December 24, 2014

Merry Christmas everyone. I hope everything works out to-night and Santa puts discharge instructions in Eric's stocking. Miss all of you in Minnesota.
—Greg Yetzer, December 24, 2014

Michelle, so glad for the good news in your update! Hope he gets to go home tomorrow! Take care of each other… bless-ings to you and your family!!!
—Kate Beverley, December 24, 2014

12-25-2015: Jesus Is Born! Eric Is Discharged!

By Eric's mom, Thursday, December 25, 2014

Merry Christmas, everyone!

Well, Eric got his Christmas wish. :) We left the hospital just after 3 p.m. and headed to Huntington Beach, where Eric prefers to spend recovery. He still has a long way to go in getting everything in sync and more comfortable, but hopefully being in his own place, in his own bed, and near his favorite beach will get things turned around.

We will head back to USC on Tuesday to see the surgeon, and hopefully the pathology report will be completed by then. If everything is clear, Eric will have his port removed and will be completely free!

Hopefully, Eric will be up to writing in a few days. If not, I will post an update Tuesday evening. We hope everyone had a wonderful Christmas and the joy continues!

Hugs all around!

Love, Mom

Favorite Comments

No place like home… great news!
—Mark Foss, December 28, 2014

Two of the best Christmas presents 1) Cancer free, and 2) Discharged to home, yippee.
—Kate Beverley, December 26, 2014

Hopefully Eric got more than coal and Red Bull this year.
—David Slifka, December 26, 2014

Glad to see Santa still visits the sick kids to fulfill their Christmas wishes. Rest up Eric!
—Brandon, December 25, 2014

Random Instagram Stuff

NO MORE CANCER
To Mr Cal.
From Ms Denmark
Christmas 2014

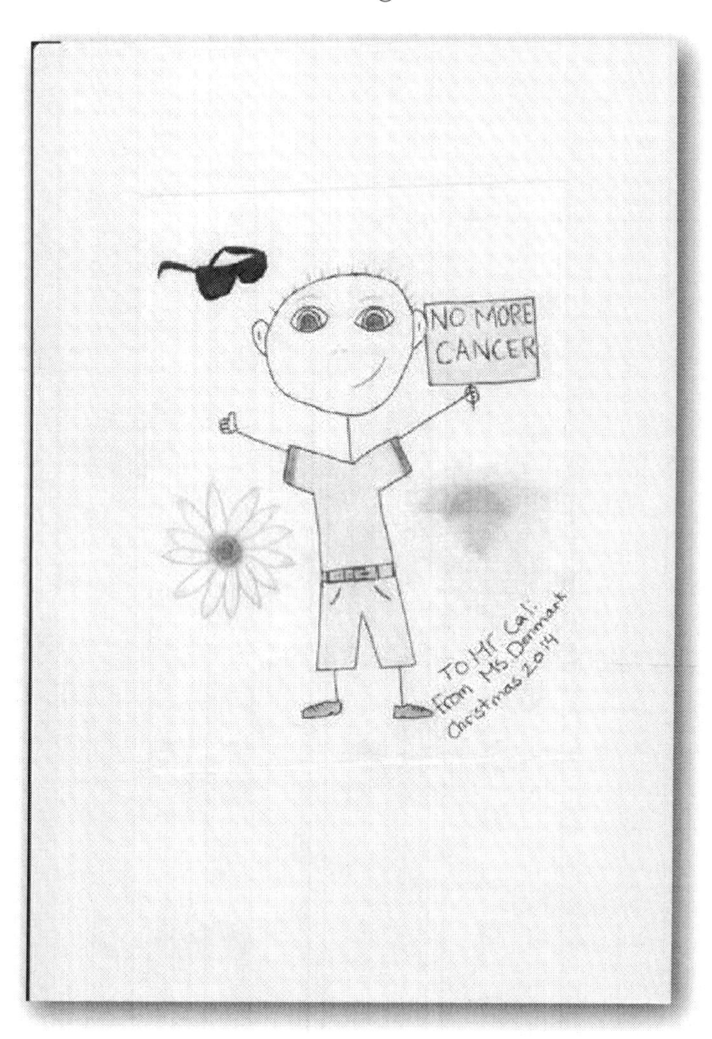

This was sent to me right after I got out of my final surgery by this adorable 18-year-old Danish girl on Instagram. @mariaegr96

12-30-2014: Officially In Remission!!

by Eric Glynn, Tuesday, December 30, 2014

We did it! Remission, y'all. Ok, ok, but back up.

So surgery was last Monday… eight days ago. All went very well. I was eating solid foods the next morning, and only had to spend three nights at the hospital. Granted, that SUCKED as the food was brutal, nurses would come in every other hour at night to draw blood or check my vitals, and I had about 900 tubes going into my stomach, back, arms and a catheter… it was a blast.

The toughest part was kickstarting my digestive system again. I had this adorable nurse a couple days in a row. Right around my age. We chatted and flirted a lot the first day and it was a fun distraction. Her name is Chlarize, so naturally that was met with, "Hello, Chlarize," in my best Hannibal Lector impersonation.

So anyway, after a couple days in the hospital, my digestive system was still in shock and all stuffed up, which is common after this surgery. But I was like, disgustingly bloated from a few days of hospital food and I wanted it OUT. So I awkwardly requested a suppository. For anyone who doesn't know what that is, it's about an inch-long cylinder… looks like a small piece of blackboard chalk… that they shove up your ass. It dissolves and helps loosen the bowels. Neat.

So I request it aaaaaand in walks cute little Chlarize, who had just started her shift. Great. I turn on my side, she puts on some gloves and rams the suppository and her finger straight on in there. She was so cool about it though. Right before she did it she says, "I feel like I should buy you dinner first…" Awesome.

The good news is the suppository worked. The bad news is I think that experience combined with her later pulling out my catheter made me shyly cower in my bed the rest of my stay, so I never asked for her number.

Moving on. I got discharged on Christmas Day, and we drove straight to Huntington Beach. The first couple days the pain and digestive stuff was very uncomfortable… I was in bed, only got up to go to the bathroom and didn't eat much. I gave MYSELF multiple suppositories. You haven't lived until you've done that. I also had to inject myself with blood thinning shots and will have to continue to do so. Nurse Eric over here.

The pain is still pretty brutal when I try to get out of bed or stand from sitting, but it's already 10 times better than on my day of discharge, and I'm eating normally now. I can walk pretty well, but at a slow pace and have to hunch over a bit, as standing up straight kind of pulls on the wound. It's gonna be one hell of a scar.

Anyway, anyway, anyway…

So today was the follow-up appointment with the surgeon to get the pathology report on the tumor and lymph nodes he removed. And per the spoiler in my journal title, we got great news! He was able to get everything out of there and the tests showed that I'm cancer free! Officially in remission! High fives all around in the clinic room, and a firm handshake, and thank you, to my surgeon, ensued.

The wound is healing up great, and it's just a matter of continuing to rest and no heavy lifting for the next eight weeks. We are still targeting an April return-to-work time frame, so there's no rush to hop back into the workforce too early or anything like that.

So, right after that clinic visit, I had a quick surgery to have the port removed from my chest. Last step, complete.

Thank you to every single person who read this blog, left a comment, sent me a text or email, gave me a call, came to visit or sent a gift or card my way during this journey. The total support was absolutely overwhelming and incredible. I so look forward to my first trip back home to Minnesota to celebrate this team victory with you all in person.

So that's it! After five surgical procedures and four cycles of chemo over four months, it's all done. 2015 is going to be alllllllll Eric, baby.

Favorite Comments

You are amazeballs... wait, maybe only amazeball? Love ya kid, can't wait to see you soon, San Francisco is always available and Salesforce.com would be lucky to have you buddy. Happy New Year to you and everyone else reading this, thinking the same thing I am… we are all so lucky and blessed to ring this new year in… love and give thanks to all yawl…

—Mark Harrison, January 1, 2015

The best news for 2015 right there! We think about you every day and send good thoughts and mojo your way. Keep kicking ass Eric!
—Liza and Kris Meacham, December 31, 2014

Wow what an incredible, positive post! Such great news, Eric. I don't think you can start off 2015 any better. Way to kick cancer's balls and leave that disease to the past year!!
—Jennifer Dixon, December 31, 2014

Best news ever!!!!!! Nothing better then answered prayers. ;) You have been blessed and given a second chance in life!!!!!! God has great plans for you, open your heart and let him show you the way!!!! 2015 is brought to you by the letter F: Freedom, Fabulous, Friends, Family, Future, Fun and getting to know your Forgiving, Faithful, Father!!!! Here's to you and second chances, cheers!!!! Loves sent,
—Cindy Weber, December 31, 2014

You just made me smile! Atta kid, Eric! Atta kid!
—Mark Foss, December 31, 2014

YOU ROCK!!!! Starting 2015 CANCER FREE!!! I knew you would kick C's you-know-what ;-) Ok, now, since you are officially in remission, it's time to spend your energy on figuring out what's going to make it all worth it... what do you WANT to do in the years to come? Who do you want to be? Where do you want to go? Who is worth investing your life into? What gifts do you have that can't go to waste?

It's yours to decide. And if you let him, God will give some wacky wonderful ideas to consider. I'm so proud of you!!!
—Wendy Housholder, December 31, 2014

Don't worry Eric, I've had that "helping hand" as well. Just part of the experience... oh, and, congratulations on the great news!
—Scott, December 30, 2014

I teared up reading your post... just what everyone has been praying for! Congrats to you Eric for fighting this beast, and BEATING it!! Give your body some time to heal and then I believe you will be a force to reckon with in this world!!
—Jill Zweber, December 30, 2014

You DO have to share your journey, Eric. You have a gift to provide humor, reality, and your mom!!! Goosebumps on your great news! Happy New Year to you and ALL of your supporters!
—Kristin Ritter, December 30, 2014

I knew you totally had it, but I'm super jacked anyway! Can't wait to celebrate and treelize... chicks dig scars.
—John, December 30, 2014

You have earned an awesome 2015! Your positive attitude is amazing. You have so many people rooting for you, because of who you are. You are grateful for life and the many blessings you've been given.
Yea, Eric!
—Patti Feldman, December 30, 2014

That is absolutely wonderful news. I am sooooo happy for you, and commend you on your strength during this journey.
—Sandy Menke, December 30, 2014

Random Instagram Stuff

LA
It could be...
It might be...
It's
GONE!
way to hit cancer out
of the ballpark!
KERSHAW
22
Dodgers

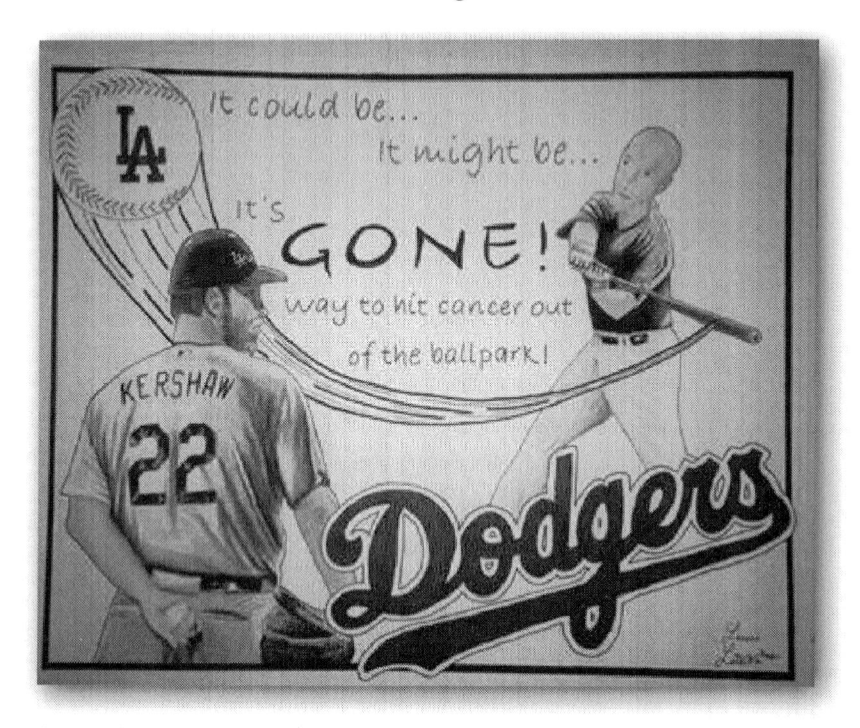

An Instagramer MAILED this to me after my surgery. She's an artist and we had a couple good conversations about personal struggles. @artistic_leanne

Random Instagram Stuff

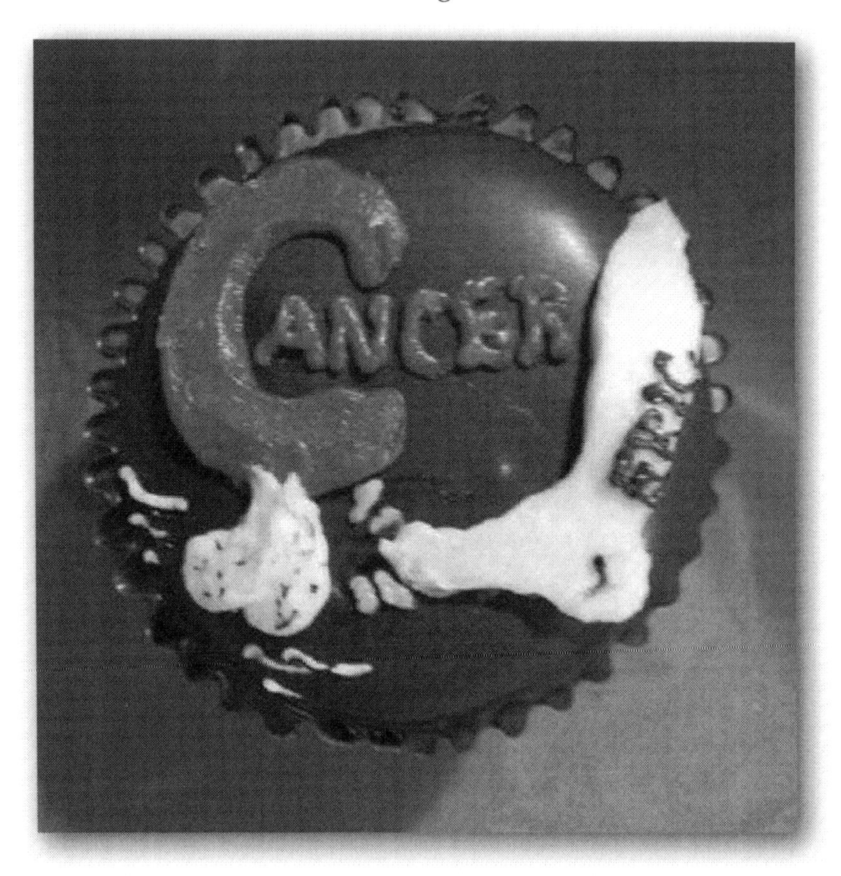

Huntington Beach cupcake-maker @sweetcakeshb made this cupcake for me, depicting me kicking cancer in the balls :)

Instagram 12-30-14 @eric_t_glynn

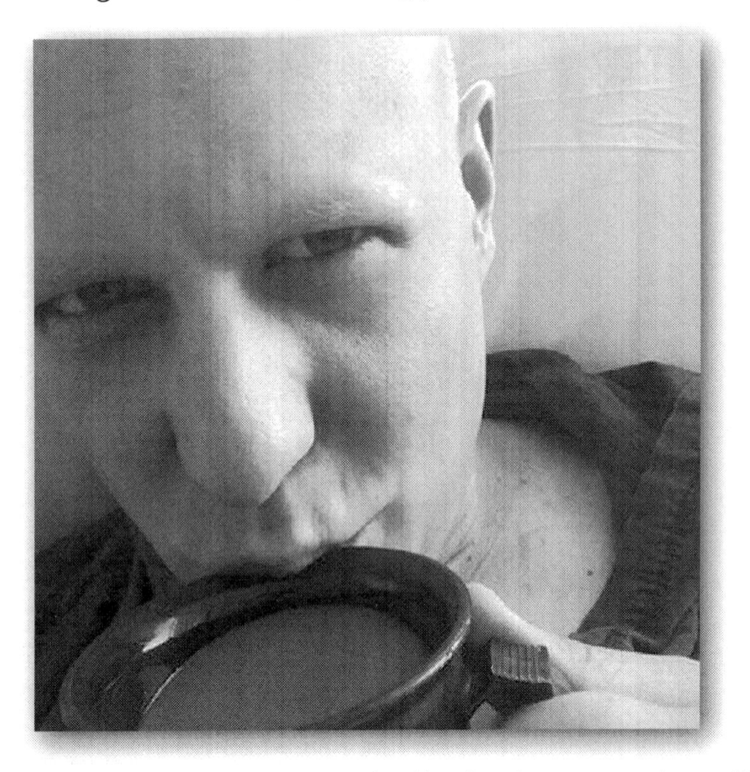

Drinking coffee with a smile on my face like a boss because...I was just notified that I'M OFFICIALLY CANCER FREE AND IN REMISSION! Surgery was a success last week and I've started the 12 week healing process. I was diagnosed on September 3rd...5 surgical procedures and 4 cycles of chemo later and I'm finally ready to hit the life restart button. 2015 is gonna be allllll Eric :) Thank you all so much for following along, leaving comments of hope, and sharing personal stories through all this. I feel that my story is just starting in many ways. I can't wait to continue to share it with you all ^_^ #douchyselfieoftheday #cancerfree #youretougherthanyouknow #fighter #cancer #chemo #support #cancersucks #instalove #loveyouguys #superbald #starttoday #fitness #workout #gym #weightlifting #fitfam #weightloss #selfie #cali #california #socal #westcoast #huntingtonbeach #hb #ca #la #losangeles

Favorite Comments

@ski***

Eric, this is wonderful!!!!! So good to hear and you can be so proud of yourself. Not only were you strong and never gave up hope, but you also inspired people around the world with your courage. So leave 2014 with a big bang and all the best for 2015. A hug from Germany.

@rri***

Congratulations!! That is absolutely amazing! :):)<3<3

@leo***

Congratulations, boy. It's been awesome to see your path being trailed with such force and positive thoughts!

@sar***

Happy New Year to you, you kicked it, yeah. Awesome! Just heard your story and must say you are such a strong fighter! Congratulations and all the best for 2015. (((hugs)))

@sbi***

Epic news. You go buddy! Happy New Year to you.

@rod***

Man, I give you all the kudos for going through all this like a boss. I had an aunt that didn't make it because her diagnosis was quite late and the disease had spread out. So congrats man, you deserve the best in life. Have a good year!!!

@cal***

2015 is going to be your year!

@dea*****
You did it! You're a beast!!! You can do anything!!! Congrats!!! <3

@con*****
I'm SOOOOO happy for you :) Many, many thanks for sharing your thoughts with us. You have been a great inspiration. I wish you ALL THE BEST in the future and will continue to follow you. Lots of love sent to you from Conny in Denmark. <3

@_pi*****
I just read your Insta, from your first picture to your last picture as you told me to. And wow. You're such a beautiful human being. How you managed to look amazing through surgery and chemo is quite an accomplishment. But more so, how you remained positive is even more impressive. Congratulations on being cancer free! Hopefully this new year keeps you that way. XOXO

@amb*****
Very #inspirational. You are very strong and your #positivity is so refreshing, especially through a tough situation. I see great things in your future!!! Keep up the good work :) <3

@mr. *****
I legit started reading the caption on this photo and I got maybe one sentence in and started bawling my eyes out, I'm so happy.

@_ju*****
Congratulations on being cancer free and in remission. Thank you for sharing your journey with us.

@cee*****

First off, way to take your cancer by the horns and beat it down to nothingness!! I've survived 2 bouts of cancer so far. I love seeing other survivors out there doing their thing!!

12-31-2014: "It Was The Best Of Times. It Was The Worst Of Times."

by ERIC'S MOM, Wednesday, December 31, 2014

Hi Everyone!

On January 29, 1986, Dr. Johansen announced, "It's a boy!" I was SO happy. I was SO proud. I was SO thankful. I was SO humbled. I was SO excited for Eric's future.

On December 30, 2014, Dr. Daneshmand announced, "It's benign!" I was SO happy. I was SO proud. I was SO thankful. I was SO humbled. And I am SO excited for Eric's future!

There are no words I could ever write to adequately thank all of you for the part you have played in Eric's past, present and future. I am so thankful to our friends (old and new), and family (old and new), all around the world. Our employers and coworkers. Eric's Huntington Beach neighbors, and all the wonderful people of Glendale and Huntington Beach. I am thankful God placed Eric back in California at just the right time, so that he could be treated at USC by the best team in the country, from the valet guys all the way up the food chain to our awesome oncologist and surgeon, and EVERYONE in between! I am thankful for this CaringBridge family, Instagram family, and Facebook family, whether you posted words of encouragement and support, or followed along and kept us in your thoughts and prayers, it all mattered and made a difference.

Above all, I am thankful to our mighty and merciful God. As I write this, my heart is so full of abundant joy for Eric, but at the same time I know there are some reading this who are right in the middle of great trial and unbearable heartache. I will keep you close in my prayers, and I ask everyone who reads this to please lift up a prayer of healing and comfort to everyone who visits this site. Amen. POL.

Finally, Eric will have an eight week follow up, a six month follow up, and a one year anniversary follow up, so we will give an update at those times. For anyone who wants to follow the research study Eric is in, you can go to clinicaltrials.gov, and type into the search: Randomized phase II trial of Paclitaxel, Ifosfamide and Cisplatin(TIP) vs. Bleomycin, Etoposide and Cisplatin (BEP). Not only is Eric the first participant at the USC site, he is the first participant assigned to the TIP arm, which is the hope for future first line testicular cancer treatment. I'm sure Eric's results have made for some very happy researchers. :) Eric also consented to their performing genetic and protein testing on the tumor to better understand how people respond to chemo to affect chemo choices for treatment, and to see if there are any genetic changes that can be linked to cancer to help understand ways to prevent, diagnose and treat cancer going forward.

Quick update! His head and upper lip hair is growing by the day... and staying attached!

Blessings to all of you in 2015! Thank you!

Hugs all around!

Love, Mom

Favorite Comments

Beautiful words from a wonderful person. I am so happy for you and your family. Have a wonderful and blessed 2015!
—Sandy Menke, January 1, 2015

Oh Shelli, none of these blessing even would have been possible without your sacrifice, knowledge, dedication and hard work!!!! Thank you for all you have given up to make sure this went as well as it did for Eric. I'm sure he is more than appreciative and thankful, and so are all of us that love you both. ;) Happy new year sister bear!!! Xxxooo
—Cindy Weber, December 31, 2014

He's not going to go all wonky with this hair thing and grow a Duck Dynasty beard is he?! Ha!
—Carrie Harpell, December 31, 2014

Stock at American Crew, Redken, and Garnier just rose 25 percent.
—David Slifka, December 31, 2014

Instagram 1-8-14 @eric_t_glynn

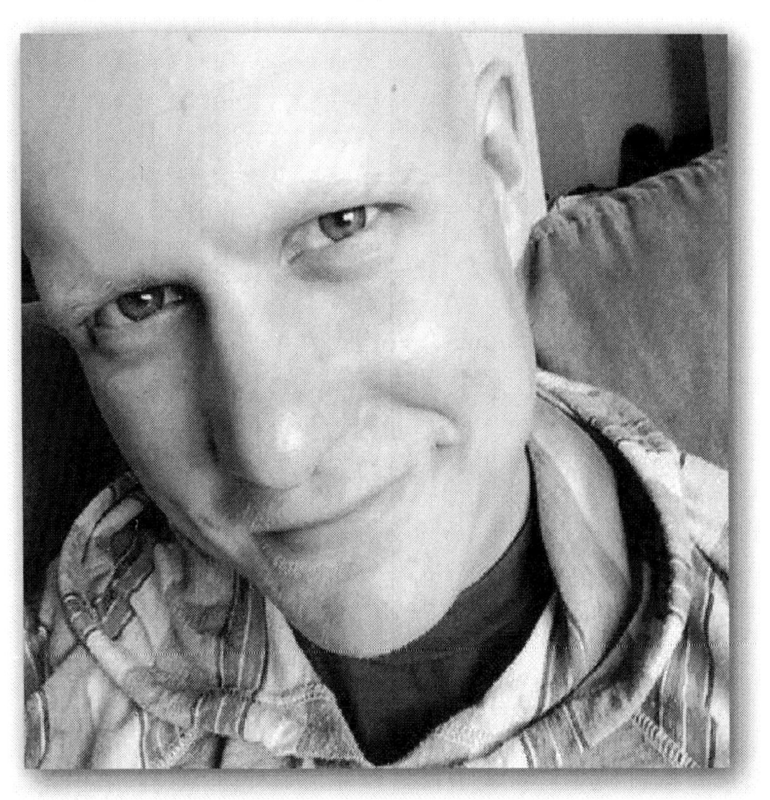

Do you see facial hair? I see facial hair! Now I just need those eyebrows... ^_^ Surgery recovery is going very well. I walk around the apartment like a grandpa but pain meds definitely help. I can't lift much more than a gallon of milk or I'll rip the stitches apparently. When I heal up a bit I'll show the scar. It's a big one! But to quote Planet of the Apes: "Don't worry, blue eyes...scars make you strong." #douchyselfieoftheday #cancerfree #youretougherthanyouknow #fighter #cancer #chemo #support #cancersucks #instalove #loveyouguys #superbald #starttoday #fitness #workout #gym #weightlifting #fitfam #weightloss #selfie #cali #california #socal #westcoast #huntingtonbeach #hb #ca #la #losangeles

Favorite Comments

@lif*****

The best will come to those who wait... soon you'll look like Paul Bunyan with all that facial hair.

@ste*****

Just read through your photos. Well done for kicking cancer's butt, sweetie! You're an inspiration to all :) It must have been gutting to get into an exercise regime and completely turn yourself around and get into shape to be told you have cancer. Wishing you a very speedy recovery! XO

@its*****

Brows or no brows, you look awesome!

@bri*****

AW YOU'RE MY FAVORITE PERSON <3

@ech*****

Eyebrows are overrated. You can always draw some :)

@jan*****

Yay! Just keep that fuzz on your face, don't drop 'em into your soup :) It's good to see you post again. #adoucheyselfieofthedaykeepsthedoctorsaway

@jol*****

Laughing and crying at the same time watching your stories. I hope you get well soon. I keep my fingers crossed :)

@hel*****

Just read through and saw all the pictures in your story. It's so incredibly inspiring and I hope all is well for you because you deserve it. It's so amazing how much it touched me, yet you live on the other side of the world. I think you have done the right thing sharing your story so you can help others through hard times too. Thank you for being the reason I smile today and whenever times get tough. Definitely following to see how your journey goes on :) <3

@mel*****

So inspirational. I hope you have a great support system. My grandmother passed away from pancreatic cancer in 2010, so this makes me hopeful for other people diagnosed with cancer. Congrats on everything though!

@rai*****

I'm so glad you made it through, with a grin nonetheless. You should write that memoir.

@fit*****

Wow, such an amazing story hun! It's such a whirlwind to go through, but health and healing is on its way. And speaking as one former cueball to another, the eyebrows do grow back, I promise! :) <3

@pan*****

I've gone through your profile twice and both times it has brought tears to my eyes! I'm so happy that you are a survivor! Stay strong! :)

@bre*****

You are in my prayers. Eric is a lovely name. It was my dad's name. He was a victim of cancer in 2010.

@kar***

YOU ARE SIMPLY AMAZING <3 Started this account for fitness progress posts, then this turned into a completely different direction and became a kicking cancer's ass account, lol! Also I really think it was a good thing you were in such good shape, but maybe it didn't matter because it was meant to be that you get cancer free! Idk... all I know is that I'm really happy for you. Stay strong, stay healthy and happy!

@via***

Wow, incredible story of pictures. You're well on your way, and you should feel very proud of yourself for all that you've accomplished. All the best of health and luck to you, friend <3 <3

@nic***

I just read through all your posts on all your pictures and I am amazed at how strong and amazing you have been through this journey! A journey that will inspire and give hope to the hopeless facing cancer treatment and the low times that it brings. I pray that 2015 is a year of much love and fullness of life, for you deserve it. Thankfully I have not been directly affected by cancer through family and friends, but your journey and testimony has given me even more hope that I can get through difficult times. Thanks for sharing!

@pac***

Wow, you're giving all cancer patients hope :)

@fit***

So handsome and inspiring. Followed your story for a while now and I'm so happy you've made it. Keep up the good work and the great attitude.

@old*****

You have such a brave fighting attitude and you are such an inspiring man. I can't wait for your eyebrows to come on back. Keep on smiling brother :) Regards from Derbyshire, England.

@_mi*****

I respect you so much for posting your journey on Instagram. I am so happy you're cancer free and you're an inspiration to us all. Your positivity is amazing and beautiful. You're so handsome too xoxo.

1-20-2015: Healin’

by ERIC GLYNN, Tuesday, January 20, 2015

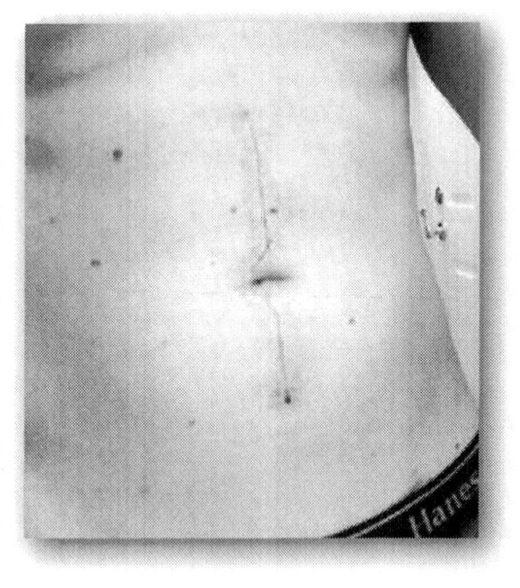

Long time no write! So… hi!

Four weeks after surgery and healing is going really well. Probably on my last couple days of pain meds. I’m walking around pretty normally… don’t look quite like a dork anymore, all hunched over. I wince a bit getting in and out of bed, and it usually takes a few steps after I wake up before I can get back to standing up straight. I posted a picture of the scar. It’s healing up quite nicely and is a lot smaller than I was expecting.

I didn’t mention it earlier, but along with the stomach surgery I also got my prosthetic silicone testicle implanted. So my ball bag is full again! I’m proud to say that I have my balance back. I will say that the ole "turn-and-cough" only has the effect on the real one, but as far as presentation goes: legit.

Oh, and there was actually a strange side-effect that could have happened because of the surgery. There was a chance that the surgeon could have nicked some tube or vessel or something, with the side-effect being that when I ejaculate, the ejaculation would go inside of my stomach instead of coming out. Super gross to think about, right? Well... have no fear... for I have "tested" it out and alllll is normal. Thumbs up.

Moving on. I have a follow-up appointment with my surgeon and chemo doctor in three weeks just to make sure all blood work is normal, and that they're pleased with my healing. At that time I'd be cleared to get back to any normal physical activity, so I'll be able to start lifting weights for the first time since September. SO excited to get back on that. I'm almost certain that I don't have an ounce of muscle on my body, so if you see me in the gym curling 5 lb dumbbells... I'm doing my best... and I'll probably also need a spotter.

I'm absolutely bored out of my mind though. I thought sleeping in, playing video games and eating pizza for three months would be fun, but I was wrong. So wrong, in fact, that I'm considering a Minnesota visit in February sometime. Don't remind me of what Minnesota weather is like, or I'll get scared and not get on the plane. But it'll be good to see family and friends. And to avoid stealing Annie's wedding thunder in April, and Mike and Kristy's wedding thunder in June.

Oh, one other kind of fun thing. I had a public relations company reach out to me and they want to help me with my book. I sent them all my CaringBridge posts and some of my favorite comments, and all of my Instagram posts and comments to see how well that could tell my story. They're editing it as we speak and after that's all put together, I'll do some narration work and hopefully have a book that the company would help pitch to publishers. And if it could lead to speaking engagements, whether they be at physician conferences, partnering up with insurance companies, student gatherings, etc., it could be a fun little way to make some money. I've always wanted to combine writing and public speaking into a career somehow. Maybe this will finally be my path.

Or maybe I get an email from the PR company tomorrow telling me I suck. Either way, it's a fun little distraction from just sitting here and staring at my TV all day.

Favorite Comments

So glad you are still posting on CaringBridge. I missed your sense of humor! That's great that you are doing so well and we are thrilled for you. Love the idea of a book and can't wait to read it! When you come back to Minnesota in February you will be such a celebrity and main attraction that you will probably have to go back to Huntington Beach just to get some rest.

—Mary Jo Jasper, January 22, 2015

Wow!! That's some scar!! What the heck happened??!! What does the other guy look like?? (LOL!! We know he's history!! Yay!!) You know you'll have to get used to answering that question... I'll get you started... you had an alien pod removed from your belly... you cut yourself shaving... you were picking the lint out of your belly button, and the lint won... you were in a knife fight... that's how you lost all that weight... you had this tattoo removed... well Harry Potter has a lightning shaped scar... you had a hangnail... you scratched a little too hard... you'll NEVER wear that giant Elvis belt buckle again... LOL!! Just a little something to make you smile since you've inspired me so much!! So glad you're on the up and up!! YOU ROCK!! Kisses to your mom...
—Helen Blythe-Hart, January 21, 2015

Eric! Such cool news! Congrats. I'm excited to hear where this may go with the PR company :) Tell them that in order for you to do the narration work, you'll need access to some resources in Paris and parts of Italy (that way they will send you here and we can hang out!)
—Chewer, January 21, 2015

You can steal my thunder Eric... it'll be hard though. ;) Come home in February! Can't believe you are gonna become the published one in the family. I thought I was going to be a poet! That is just awesome. Woot woot. Love you.
—Anne Yetzer, January 21, 2015

That Winston Churchill quote? "If you are going through hell..." This is what the other side looks like.

Atta kid.
—Mark Foss, January 21, 2015

Looking good, Eric. One way to keep muscling through it is to keep in mind that all the wincing, stooping, and hunched-over walking is great practice for when you're an old man… like me.
—MarkRisa Palony, January 21, 2015

Wow, your scar looks great!!!! So nice to hear from you and even more happy that you're doing so well ;) The gym will feel good I'm sure and knowing you, you'll be up to 10 lb presses in no time. ;)
—Cindy Weber, January 21, 2015

Personally I was really hoping for a jagged scar. You know something that looked like you were in a sword fight or a knife fight like in the "Beat It" music video. Then you could tell people it was an accident while being an extra on the set of Game of Thrones, or that the ghost of Michael Jackson stabbed you.
—Justin McMartin, January 21, 2015

I am thinking a Minnesota visit sounds grand... people to see and hug, practice speaking to groups to see it you really like it, let your mom show off her wonder boy and then appreciate the California weather even more when you return... LOL.
—Roxy McGraw, January 20, 2015

Wow. Daneshmand does an awesome job. Do you think there is love in every stitch? I am so glad you are doing well and may come to visit in February. I think I saw on our BCBSMN Intranet that there is a take-your-cancer-free-kid-to-work-day in February. ;)

Honestly, there are so many who just want to see you and hug on you and wish you continued healing, Eric. Come home.

I miss you. Love, Mom

—Eric's mom, January 20, 2015

Instagram 1-21-14 @eric_t_glynn

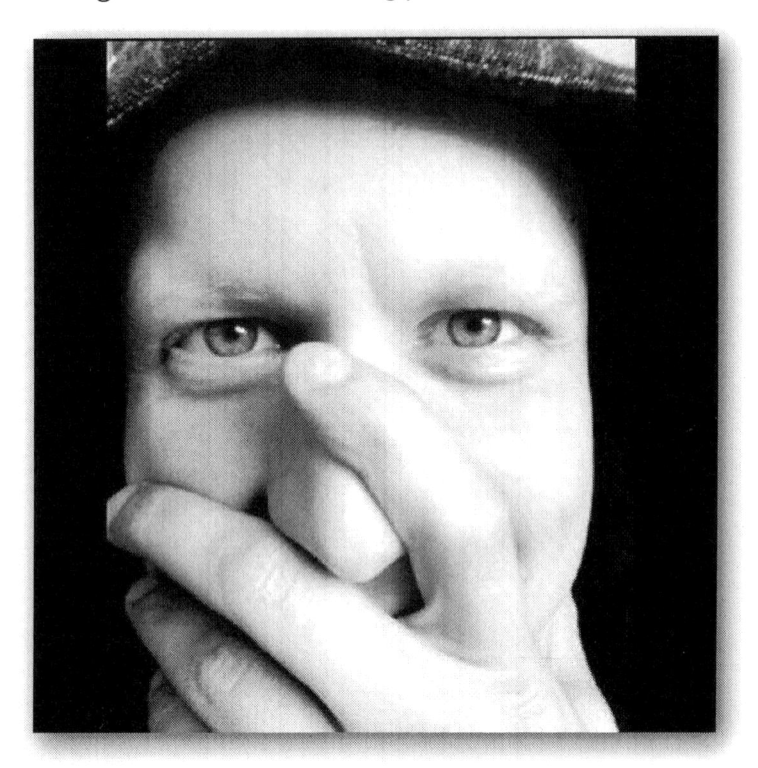

I'm seriously so blown away by the number of messages, shoutouts and DMs I get daily. It really shows how amazing people are. Today is the first day I can do cardio! Lifting starts in 3 weeks. I'm so excited to put cancer behind me and get back to my first love: fitness. I'll track my progress here...not too excited about posting the 'before' shots aka today but when I have something to compare it to then it'll be better. And when it's healed up enough I'll show off my big scar! #douchyselfieoftheday #cancerfree #youretougherthanyouknow #fighter #cancer #chemo #support #cancersucks #instalove #loveyouguys #superbald #starttoday #fitness #workout #gym #weightlifting #fitfam #weightloss #selfie #cali #california #socal #westcoast #huntingtonbeach #hb #ca #la #losangeles

Favorite Comments

@mud***

I thought I was your first love <3

@bri***

Eyeballs :) <3

@jed***

Can I just say how awesome it is that you're cancer free?! Cancer is a bitch.

@gal***

You are awesome and your eyes look like the world.

@23t***

Awesome selfie!!!! :) <3 Enjoy your cardio...

@sma***

Just keep that amazing light in your eyes! Lots of love! Can't wait to see all the gains you will make quickly.

@mr_***

Hey! I'm really glad that you've reached the end of your journey! I went through the same thing that you did. I was told I didn't have cancer anymore on 1/7/2015... so just a few days after you! I'm glad we both won the battle :) If you don't mind me asking, what kind of cancer did you have? I had bone cancer in my right shoulder.

@mal***

I'm so happy for you! God bless! Support all the way from Cairo, Egypt!!

@jes***

Good for you!!!!! Breast cancer runs in my family and I absolutely love seeing somebody who doesn't let cancer run their life!!!! I admire you so much <3

@lou***

Sending you love and support all the way from Malaysia! You are such an inspiration. Your story made me realize how I am blessed and full of God's grace. Will pray for you, that you will recover ASAP!! God bless :)

@loo***

I'm so proud of you! Your fighting spirit and positivity touched my heart... stay strong!!

@cyp***

I started at the bottom and worked my way up to your most recent pic. I noticed many changes, but the one thing that I noticed never changed, was the look in your eyes. You always, even in the chemo pics, had the sparkle and light in those eyes. Stay strong, get stronger and heal fast! And btw, cancer sucks!!! Good luck!!

@dor***

You are inspirational! I feel like God had an amazing plan for your brand new life! It's like you had a rebirth! Go and do whatever and just enjoy it!

@pan***

Much appreciated :) They say "Fall in love with someone's eyes because the eyes never age," but in your case they never changed. Your weight loss, your illness, your recovery... no matter how you changed physically, always the same eyes. But seriously you're an extremely positive man and that's refreshing in this day and age. I spent two months dieting and exercising only to give it up once I felt secure with my body and of course I went straight back to undoing all that work, but you kept going and that's the motivation I needed and the lesson I've learned – don't quit while you're ahead.

Instagram 1-30-2015 @eric_t_glynn

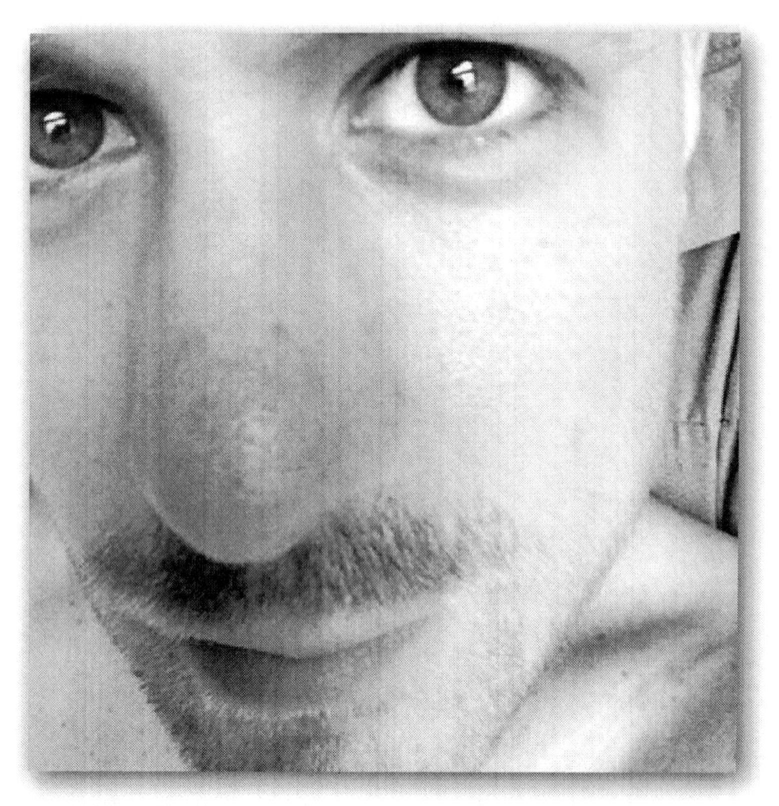

Aaaand I'm officially 29 today. Something tells me 29 is going to be a bit better than 28! I've been able to lift weights and do cardio for a week now. Feels so good to move around. Granted, I get a crazy side ache about 200 calories into cardio and can only lift half the weight I used to for each exercise, but it'll be fun to grow my strength and stamina back. Maybe someday soon I'll be IG shirtless again! #douchyselfieoftheday #cancerfree #youretougherthanyouknow #fighter #cancer #chemo #support #cancersucks #instalove #loveyouguys #superbald #starttoday #fitness #workout #gym #weightlifting #fitfam #weightloss #selfie #cali #california #socal #westcoast #huntingtonbeach #hb #ca #la #losangeles

Favorite Comments

@the***

Happy birthday, and your stash is looking good!

@flo***

Happy Bday! From a Venezuelan girl <3 <3 <3

@jus***

Happy birthday!!!!!!!! #staystrong

@fit***

Happy birthday handsome! So proud of you for pushing through what had to be one of the hardest years of your life. Wishing you a happy, healthy, amazing year, and many more to come <3

@eny***

Happy birthday! I know you've had it rough so you truly deserve a fantastic birthday with many more to come! :)

@mis***

I've seen all your Instapics. You are amazing, a very good example of life! Happy birthday darling, good vibes!!!

@ang***

Those beautiful eyes... so full of life. Happy birthday and may the next year (and all the rest of your many years) bring you nothing but happiness and joy.

@spe***

Happy birthday babe!! You're so strong, it's inspirational! And I don't know how you've kept that positive attitude throughout your whole journey… you're truly incredible!! I hope this year is spectacular for you. I hope you can get to your fit goal and weight goal and health goal. You should just reach all your goals and be successful without losing your positive attitude and incredible outlook on life. You're so amazing and inspirational!! I'm so happy you're pulling through! It was an honor to watch you grow and continue to watch you grow through this journey!! Love you babe! Happy birthday! :)

@bee***

Looking forward to shirtless IG photos. Happy birthday XOXO

@xin***

My mum is cancer free and just celebrated her bday yesterday! Every year will be better than the previous! Press on! I admire you guys so so much! Congratulations and happy birthday!

@cho***

Happy belated birthday, babe! I wish I could spank you!!! Hahaha…

Instagram 2-2-2015 @eric_t_glynn

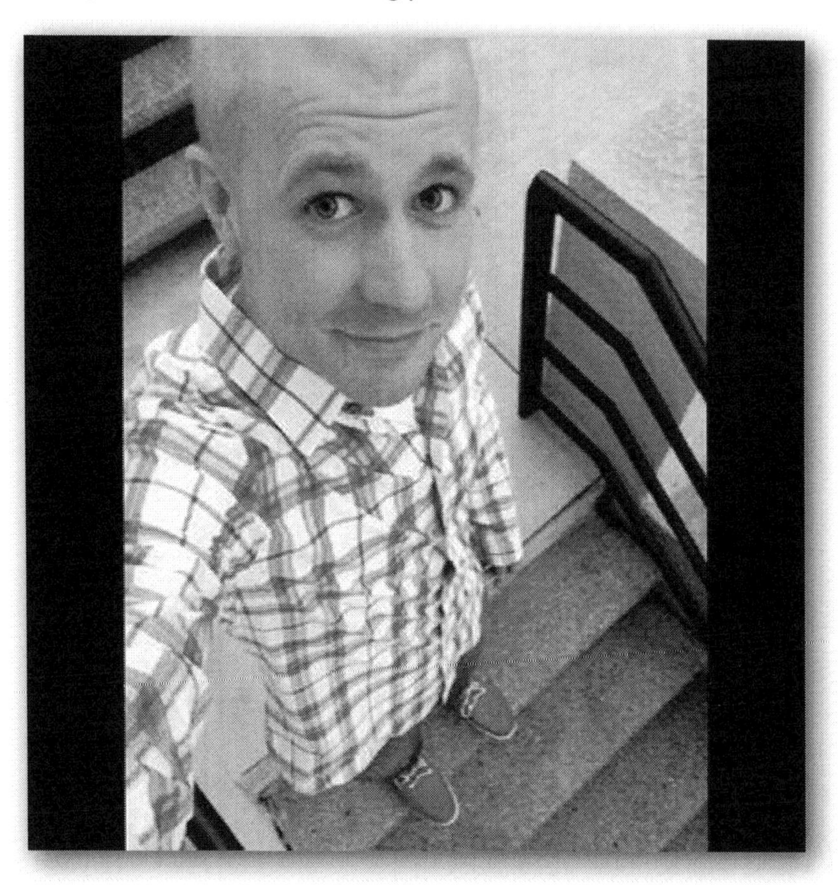

I wore a dress shirt for the first time in 5 months over the weekend. Finally getting back to my preppy roots ^_^ Looking less and less like a bald ghost every day! It's so exciting to be blasting through the light at the end of the tunnel. The sunshine is on my face and it feels gooooooood. #douchyselfieoftheday #cancerfree #youretougherthanyouknow #fighter #cancer #chemo #support #cancersucks #instalove #loveyouguys #superbald #starttoday #fitness #workout #gym #weightlifting #fitfam #weightloss #selfie #cali #california #socal #westcoast #huntingtonbeach #hb #ca #la

Favorite Comments

@add***

This is by far my fav Instagram account, you should DM ME!

@miv***

Yyyyyyiiiihhhhaaaaa!!! You look great!!! Glad for you! :)

@kri***

Looking great! So refreshed, love it.

@iva***

You look so great! Sending lots of positive vibrations your way! <3 <3 Your story is very inspiring.

@kit***

Lookin' good Eric! My dad is starting his fight today. You have been an inspiration.

@fre***

I love your story and your positivity. Thank you for sharing it. #strongwill. You're the man! Keep it up.

@ret***

Loving that turquoise!!!! You rock it!!!! :D

@nqd***

Your Sperry collection, haha. Happy late birthday. I'm sorry I didn't call.

@jun***

Glad to see you're feeling better. FYI, your cancer surviving date happens to be my bday :)

@swe***

WOW ~ your life path has been amazing! I am glad you are better. Keep sharing your story. People need to hear it so they can approach life more. You are inspiring! :)

@inv***

Great dude. You are now a beacon of light for others. Keep shining.

@vco***

Have just sobbed reading your mum's blog entries. Keep fighting you incredible chap! Sending much love over the pond XXX

@fra***

The perspective is really... creepy :D Your head looks so big and the rest, tiny :D

@j_m***

Love that you are documenting your journey as you battle cancer. So glad to see you have come out on top!! I was diagnosed in Nov. 2014 with stage 4 colon cancer. A few days later, my fiancé and my parents trucked my butt up to Cleveland Clinic (about a 3 hour drive from home). I was in horrible pain. Couldn't stand up straight, let alone walk. Every pothole felt like a stab. I had a 2 inch mass as well as my left ovary removed. I am proud to say as of January 2015 I am cancer free! Still taking the chemo though to make sure there isn't anything in there that they just can't see yet. You are an inspiration! I am also documenting my journey as I go through #chemo... feel free to follow.

@che***

I'm so happy for you! I hope the sunshine keeps your heart warm and that all this wonderful energy you're exuding never dims!

@suz***

You look good, babe! That color looks great on you.

@mon***

You look really good!!!! And the smile on your face is like sunshine.

2-17-2015 : Final Cancer Blog Post! :)

by ERIC GLYNN, February 17, 2015

Healthy Eric in the houuuusseeee!

Hi all. I'm doing great. It's been almost two months since the final surgery. I'm basically pain free at this point. All the scars are a bit tender to the touch, but they haven't kept me from lifting weights and doing the elliptical for the last couple of weeks. I'm already feeling a lot stronger, but I still have a long way to go. I'm eating well, moving around well. I've basically been living like a college kid on summer break the last four weeks. Staying up way too late, sleeping in way too late, eating frozen pizza and playing video games. I basically feel normal.

The hair is growing in well! I have eyebrows again, so I look far less creepy than before. My facial hair is growing in thicker than before and there's far more than peach fuzz on my head at this point. It's actually long enough to where I wake up with bed-head again. I don't think anyone has ever been so happy to have bed-head.

I have been bored out of my mind, though. To mix it up, I went up to San Francisco last week to visit friends and see Aunt Lisa, Uncle Clifford and Bryan. We had brunch overlooking the Bay Bridge, I got a free movie at Bryan's theater, and took a top-down ride in Lisa and Clifford's new BMW M4 convertible. I was never able to take that Ferrari ride like I wanted to, but this was an awesome consolation victory ride. Clifford gunned it up and down the hilly streets of SF and we gave it a couple top speed runs on the freeway. It was perfect convertible weather and it felt so good to have my "hair" blow in the wind.

I'm also headed to Minnesota tomorrow! I'll be home for a week, visiting family and friends. It's supposed to be a high of 6 degrees tomorrow. That sounds awful. Why am I going home again? Why do you all still live in Minnesota again? What is wrong with you all?

Anyway, I had my final appointment with my surgeon this morning. All blood work is normal, x-rays normal, and I got the ok to go be a normal kid. Though I've been breaking the rules and have been working out, I now officially have the ok to do so. I've also been cleared to return to work at the end of my long-term disability that goes through March. So... yay! I don't have to deal with cancer stuff anymore! I'll just have blood work and CT scans done every three months to confirm that everything is all clean and clear. But besides that, I can go back to a normal life.

Finally, my book. It's about 90 percent done! We just need to go through some more edits, clean it up, shoot a book cover and it will be ready to rock. When all is said and done, it'll be in the 190-200 page range, so it's, like, a real book! We'll be pitching it to publishers, but I'm also seriously considering just self-publishing it, or at least self- publishing it at first. After the book is completed and we have some copies in our hands, my PR team and I will reach out to CA and MN media to see if we can line up some interviews and do some publicity. And if this could all lead to speaking engagements or something like that, it would be amazing. That will be my focus the month of March… to see where that goes. If it goes nowhere, I'll head back into the software sales field, but if it picks up steam at all, I'd love to be the face of testicular cancer and speak at conferences, schools, etc. I'll keep you all posted on that as my book finishes up. We're estimating that by March we will start printing books and make them available on Amazon and other online retailers, and have electronic copies available for tablets. It's all very exciting and a fun way to pass my time as I heal.

So, that's all for me. Months ago in a blog post I said I was looking forward to the day when this blog would be done. When I could say I won and I could be a success story. Well today is finally the day. Chemo and surgeries done. Clean bill of health. Cancer free. I can officially pick up my life where I left it on September 3rd when I got diagnosed. It was only five months ago, but in many ways it has felt like five years. And almost all for the better. I have such a different outlook on life and on people. And it's because of you all. Thank you all for everything.

So that's it for this chapter of my life. I get to come home to MN to celebrate (and freeze my newly healthy balls off) and then go about my new path. I'm excited to see where it leads.

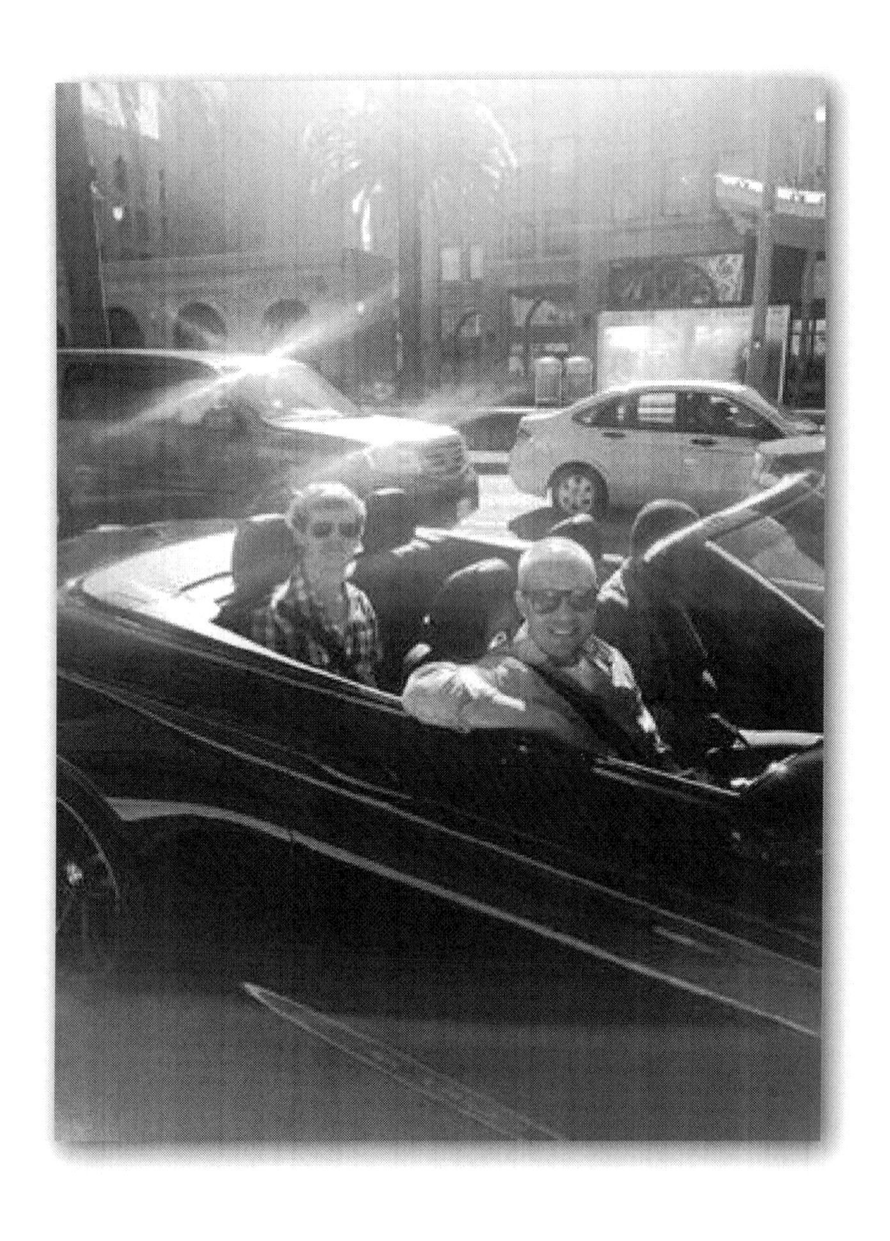

Favorite Comments

Minnesota can't wait to welcome you to it's flippin' frigid, warm-hearted state, Eric! Thanks for the update - rejoicing for you and your whole family. I will be one of the first to purchase AND promote your book young man! Mucho blessings, Kristin
—Kristin Ritter, February 18, 2015

13 below right now Eric, bring warm clothes!
—Liza and Kris Meacham, February 18, 2015

I'm so happy for you on all counts!! Yay!! I know your inspirational story will lift the spirits of others on a grand scale. Salut!!
—Helen Blythe-Hart, February 17, 2015

It's so great to hear you are doing AMAZING!!! I am excited to hear what's next in your life and wish you the best on your book deal! Your mom must be elated to have you back home for a visit!!!
—Kathy Hallblade, February 17, 2015

The face of testicular cancer? So you want to look like balls? Seriously though, congrats man. I can't imagine the trials and tribulations you went through, the pain and agonizing suffering, and downright bad times. Glad you're on the other side.
—David Slifka, February 17, 2015

How wonderful it is to hear you talk about THESE things!!!! Normal things!! Yay!! So glad to hear all the good news!! Can't wait to see you!! I love you
—Aunt Amy, February 17, 2015

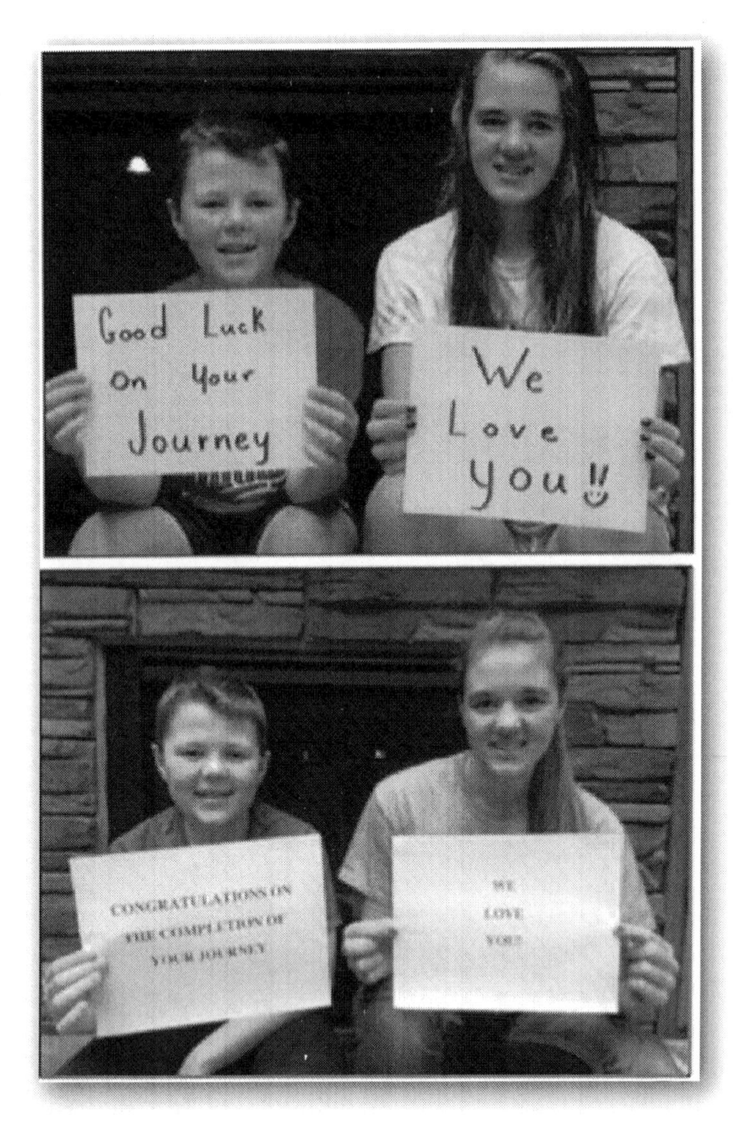

My little sister, Brianna, and brother, Garrett. The top pic was right before my first day of chemo and the bottom was after getting the "all clear" from the doctors. Love you guys :) :) :)

And So It Ends

During my battle, people told me I was inspirational. Family, friends, random Instagram users. Over and over. And while I was happy because inspiring people is wonderful, it was so often met with me shrugging my shoulders. I guess it's hard for me to grasp it. I got cancer and I took the steps to beat it. That's all I did. I truly think the only reason I was able to take it on with flare was because of the support around me. I was just being myself… the way people supported me was the inspirational part.

When I was first diagnosed, my plan was to take it on as quietly as I could. I had a small group of less than 10 people that I was updating in a private email chain and I asked them to keep it to themselves. I had a touch of a negative outlook on people in general. I was never one to get excited over big family gatherings, to hear about what's new in my extended family's lives. I had a small, close-knit group of friends, and was really close with my immediate family. And I was happy with that. I enjoyed the loner life I had the first time I lived in California and was kind of excited about more of that when I moved back out here.

But the support has absolutely blown me away. Family and friends that I never really bothered to invest time into came out of nowhere. They were constant commenters on my blog and sent texts to check-in with me all the time.

People have asked me if this whole experience has changed me. When friends came to visit in the middle of my battle, they were surprised that I hadn't changed much at all. I'm still the same sarcastic, weird goof. This was all just a little bump in the road for me.

The only thing that changed is my outlook on people. That people step up and give you strength when you are weak, perseverance when you want to quit, well-received company when you think you want to be alone. If I sat here and thanked everyone individually who helped me in some way... let's just say this book would be twice as long. You all know who you are. So this is for all of you: THANK YOU!

There are a couple people that I do want to thank individually, though.

Tony and Hallie Caracciolo. My parents met these two in France the week I was diagnosed. By coincidence, fate, or as my mom would call it, a "Godincidence," these two ended up playing a huge role in my journey, as they had a vacant apartment just minutes from USC that they generously let mom and I stay at for the 12 weeks of chemo. To open up their home to someone they had just met a couple weeks earlier was just... incredible.

An anonymous thank you is in order as well. When I was first diagnosed and knew I'd be leaving work and put on disability, I knew that I wouldn't be able to afford my Huntington Beach apartment, so all the stressors of breaking my lease and moving everything into storage while I fought cancer just added to the stress of, well, fighting cancer. But he-or-she-who-will-not-be-named swooped in and gave me the gift of getting to keep the apartment. To keep the comfort of a home for when I was healthy enough to rest up there in between chemo treatments for alone time. To have a happy place and to feel some stability. A place I could bring mom so she could go on her daily walks along the beach and meet all the Huntington Beach people who are close to me. There's no way I could ever explain how important that was and how thankful I am for this gift.

There was one more person to thank… hmm… let's see. Oh yeah, now I remember. The one who played the biggest role of all. I lovingly call her "Mudder." My mom.

She was able to go on leave from work and was with me every day of my battle. From my testicular surgery in September, every day of chemo and my final surgery on her birthday, December 22, she was by my side. There was literally no way I could have gotten through it all without her.

She made me burgers and eggs at the oddest times of the day and night when I was up for food during chemo weeks. She held my hand as we'd walk into the USC day clinic for chemo when I was frail and dizzy and close to passing out. She didn't just drop me off for chemo and go about her day. She was in the room every single day, mostly sitting in silence (at my request), becoming an expert in technology, as she'd text and email family and friends with updates on my health.

She was my drill sergeant on the days when I felt too weak to get up, too weak to eat anything. She'd sneak into my room multiple times every night to make sure I was still breathing and refill my glass of water.

She was my nurse and personal assistant. Waking me to take my medications, taking the lead with everything insurance and bill-related. She had a dozen different folders and notebooks tracking it all in a cancer suitcase that she'd carry with her every day. She was on the phone with nurses and pharmacies and insurance companies for hours and hours so that I was getting everything I needed.

Our drive to USC every day was about 20-30 minutes and we had a "Kick Cancer In The Balls" playlist that we'd play. Every day. The same songs. Some of them she chose to be in the list, some I chose. When I hear them today I think about those rides. How awful I felt but how high-spirited she always was. We'd sing along to the songs when we were both feeling ok, or she'd hum them on her own when I was having a bad day. A couple that I will never forget:

-"Glorious Unfolding," Steven Curtis Chapman (Always the first song on the playlist. Mom's choice)
-"Keep Your Head Up," Andy Grammer (My theme song through all of this. Also an excellent music video worth checking out)
-"Money On My Mind," Sam Smith (I'd sing "Mudder" on my mind, instead of "Money." It always made her laugh)
-"Shake It Off," Taylor Swift (A song I absolutely hated, but she loved)

She was the reason I was able to do my treatment in California. I would have had to pack up and move back to Minnesota after my first cycle of chemo, because it was just too intense and I was too worthless those weeks. For anyone who thinks they can do multiple cycles of week-long chemo treatments on their own... you are crazy. I needed someone by my side through it all.

Thank you so much, Mudder. I needed you. I love you.

If you take away anything from this book, take away that you shouldn't face tough times on your own. Whether it be your own cancer battle or some other health issue, a loss of a loved one, getting laid off at work, a tough breakup… people will be there to hold your hand through it. Don't be stubborn and try and face it alone. It's amazing what outside support can do for your head and your heart.

But also take away that you can handle any battle. That you can face it, and that there will be better days. To quote the Andy Grammer song from our playlist, "Only rainbows after rain, the sun will always come again."

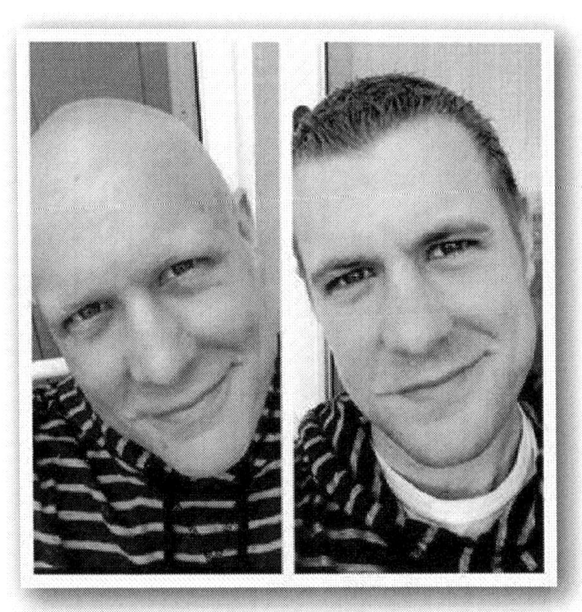

Never forget: You're stronger than you know.

Made in the USA
Lexington, KY
29 April 2015